Praise for the First Edition

You Don't LOOK Sick! is a poignant and easy-to-read journey of a person afflicted with a chronic illness, her struggle to come to terms with her disease, and her acceptance of and adaptation to it. Joy Selak takes this journey with her physician who adds to the book valuable reflection and a medical perspective. This book combines the difficult lessons learned with humor and with more grace than I could imagine mustering. This text will be very helpful to many of my patients going on the same journey.

Bob Crittenden, MD, MPH
Chief of Family Medicine
Harborview Medical Center
Seattle, Washington

This book is a masterful, insightful, and useful account of the patient's and physician's perspective, in their own words and frames of mind, on recognizing, confronting and dealing with chronic illness. This multifaceted perspective is one with which not only patients with chronic illnesses of any nature, but also their health care providers and family members, will certainly identify, and from which all will benefit. Chronic illnesses are greatly underrecognized and undertreated, and books such as this contribute to educating a broad audience in a meaningful and practical way.

Roberto Patarca-Montero, MD, PhD, HCLD
Author of *Concise Encyclopedia of Chronic Fatigue Syndrome*

If you live with a chronic condition and know others who are challenged by such a condition, this is an easy-to-understand, practical and compassionate book that shows a patient and physician partnership in healing. Many conditions cannot be cured, but all suffering can find meaning when the mind is taken seriously, the body finds balance and the spirit integrates the experience in a movement toward wholeness. Joy Selak, with the help of her physician, comes to terms with a life that is radically challenged by that process.

Hannah O'Donoghue, CCVI, RN, MS
Holistic Nurse Practitioner
Seton Cove Spirituality Center
Austin, Texas

Readers Praise *You Don't Look Sick!*

Thank you, thank you, thank you. I came across your book quite by accident in an online catalogue because the title grabbed me. Even as I clicked "place hold" I thought, here we go again, another pile of blah, blah, preaching...take this, do that, and you'll be cured, that will inevitably leave me feeling frustrated and depressed for being the only one who can't cure myself. I brightened when I saw that it was light enough to hold, propped on pillows, while I lie on the heating pad... I read excerpts from the beginning to (my husband) Willy and we looked at each other, stunned. It was like reading about our lives. I have been there and he has watched, helplessly, feeling my pain.

— Deborah Hall, London, Ontario, Canada

I ordered your book and read it in 24 hours. Thank you. It is the first of many steps I hope to be making in learning how to live well despite my chronic illness. Your book has given me some new insights and much validation. I wanted you to know.

— Sarah F. Brownell, Laredo, TX

I can't tell you how wonderful it was to read your book. I have felt everything you discussed, every feeling you were so wonderfully able to put words to. I have struggled with putting it all into words that represent my life with Sjogren's syndrome. Thank you for sharing so much with me. You have changed my life.

— Deborah Gowrie, Old Saybrook, CT

I want to thank you for taking the time, stepping out of your box and sharing your gift in your book—You Don't LOOK Sick!

— Deb M-S

You came to speak, at one of our meetings, and I remember your talk very well, and learned a lot from it. I have your book and learned a lot from that, too.

— Kari Cain, Austin, TX

I love your book and I am passing it around like a plate of mashed potatoes to everyone that knows me. It's SO helpful and explains SO much!! Next on my list, my pain management doc. She can be a real pill but is willing to listen. I hope she will read it!!

— Tracy Rupp, Atlanta, GA

On our drive home from the conference, I read your book and can relate to your experience on so many levels. The book made me laugh, cry, and mostly nod in agreement. I really feel I was meant to read this book.

— Alyssia Ventura

Thank you for writing your book. Since being diagnosed with Interstitial Cystitis and Fibromyalgia I have read everything on the subject of chronic illness that I could get my hands on. Your book is by far the most informative, enjoyable and uplifting book I have read.

— Jenny Greiner, San Juan Capistrano, CA

You Don't LOOK Sick!

Living Well with Invisible Chronic Illness

Second Edition

Joy H. Selak

and

Steven S. Overman, MD

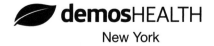 **demos**HEALTH

New York

Visit our website at www.demoshealth.com

ISBN: 978-1-936303-42-7
e-book ISBN: 978-1-617051-38-8

Acquisitions Editor: Noreen Henson
Compositor: diacriTech

Medical information provided by Demos Health, in the absence of a visit with a health care professional, must be considered as an educational service only. This book is not designed to replace a physician's independent judgment about the appropriateness or risks of a procedure or therapy for a given patient. Our purpose is to provide you with information that will help you make your own health care decisions.

The information and opinions provided here are believed to be accurate and sound, based on the best judgment available to the authors, editors, and publisher, but readers who fail to consult appropriate health authorities assume the risk of injuries. The publisher is not responsible for errors or omissions. The editors and publisher welcome any reader to report to the publisher any discrepancies or inaccuracies noticed.

Library of Congress Cataloging-in-Publication Data
CIP data is available from the Library of Congress.

Special discounts on bulk quantities of Demos Health books are available to corporations, professional associations, pharmaceutical companies, health care organizations, and other qualifying groups. For details, please contact:

Special Sales Department
Demos Medical Publishing, LLC
11 West 42nd Street, 15th Floor
New York, NY 10036
Phone: 800-532-8663 or 212-683-0072
Fax: 212-941-7842
E-mail: rsantana@demosmedpub.com

Printed in the United States of America by Bang Printing.
12 13 14 15 / 5 4 3 2 1

For Dan, again and always.

&

For Holly, who nurtures mind, body, and spirit.

We have been motivated by the feedback we have received from many chronically ill patients in Dr. Overman's offices, at conferences, and in our daily lives. We also appreciate those readers we do not know, but who found us by letter or email and took the time to tell us their stories.

Our thanks to our agent Stephany Evans at FinePrint Literary Management and Noreen Henson at Demos Health Publishing for taking on this second edition. It has been empowering to work with such consummate professionals. Our guest contributor, Bob Crittenden, MD, is valuable for his friendship, his efforts to bring about national health care reform, and his continued efforts to help those who live with chronic illness find their own path to living well.

Others who gave valuable advice and insight for this edition are: Alice Acheson, Susan Asplund, Claudia Cerenzie, Randolph "Huey" Houston, Mavourneen McGinty, Leslie Savage, Lisa Sterling, Lynne Tredennick, and Don Uslan.

Contents

Phase II: Being Sick

Phase III: Grief and Acceptance

Phase IV: Living Well

Preface to the Second Edition

You Don't LOOK Sick! Living Well with Invisible Chronic Illness was published by The Haworth Press in 2005 and we have been gratified by its success. It was a finalist for USABookNews Best Health Book that year, coming in second to *Supersize Me*. It was also runner-up for the Independent Publishers Book Awards, or IPPY, as the Best Health Book of the Year. *You Don't LOOK Sick!* became our publisher's bestseller and soon we began receiving invitations to speak at physician and patient meetings and conferences across the United States and even abroad. These in-person engagements have given us the opportunity to share our hopeful message—that it is possible to live well, even if you can't get well—to thousands who might benefit.

We have learned from our audiences and the many kind readers who took the time to send us letters. You have asked questions, shared your own stories of the challenges of invisible chronic illness, and let us know how our book helped you move forward. We also learned that our book could be better. For this edition, Joy felt she could reorganize and add to her stories so they fit the phases more accurately, and she wanted to clarify the positive opportunities that occur in even the most frustrating experiences with illness. Dr. Overman wanted to offer readers specific travel tips for each phase of the journey in order to deepen understanding and offer helpful tools to progress through the phases.

Most importantly we decided that we needed to include a fourth phase of the chronic illness experience: *Grief and Acceptance*. We had shared with readers how we learned to navigate three phases, *Getting Sick*, *Being Sick*, and *Living Well*, but this necessary additional passage, which includes grief at the loss of function, followed by acceptance that the illness is not going to go away, usually occurs first sometime near the end of the *Being Sick* phase and is likely to recur repeatedly throughout the illness journey. This time of transition allows patients to make peace with their new reality and affords the foundation and the freedom to build a new and meaningful life.

In 2007, our publisher was bought by a large British house and, soon after, the U.S. offices were closed and all operations moved to the U.K. Pricing and shipping issues with our new publisher made the continued sales success of our book in the United States impossible. We are grateful to FinePrint Literary Management and Demos Health Publishing for taking us on and believe this improved second edition will be of value to both new and returning readers.

We originally chose our stories from a collection of Joy's true life experiences that we felt were common to many with invisible illness. From a stack of ideas written on dozens of index cards, we settled on the twelve we felt best represented our three phases. For this second edition, there are still twelve stories, divided among the four phases. Some are new stories, some extensively edited, and all supported by the enhanced comments by Dr. Overman, based on the years of experience he has working with patients as they move through the phases of chronic illness.

Finally, we believe we have more avenues to help patients and health care workers cope with chronic illness successfully. We are collecting stories and strategies from patients, physicians, other practitioners, and researchers to help readers access the many, many ways they can weave a web of wellness in their lives. We look forward to offering returning readers other voices, wisdom, and experience beyond our own and activities that can support success.

Please let us hear from you and perhaps join you in person at your next meeting or conference to continue the conversation about *You Don't LOOK Sick! Living Well with Invisible Chronic Illness.*

Joy H. Selak and Dr. Steven S. Overman

Joy may be reached at joy@joywrites.com and Dr. Overman at DocOverman@gmail.com.

More information about the book can be found at: www.chronicinvisibleillness.com and www.joywrites.com

An Introductory Conversation

D r. Overman and I have some real life stories and a few simple principles we want to share with you in the coming pages. Our book isn't long, or hard to understand, and we wrote it this way on purpose. We know many of you are tired and hurting, and may be frustrated and angry that illness has robbed you of the person you once were. If your illness is invisible, you may have found it hard to find the right doctor, and you may receive little support, even suspicion, about your symptoms from friends and family. We identify and sympathize with all of this and believe you will find parts of your own life in our stories. We hope you will laugh some and maybe cry a little but, most of all, we hope you will be encouraged that the future can be better for you, even if you can't make your illness go away.

Dr. Overman and I know that our voices are specific to our own experiences and we have had many advantages, both personal and professional. However, our combined years of experience and our trial by fire as patient and physician have taught us to appreciate the diversity of the human experience that we believe will allow our book to have meaning for those with different demographics. We believe we all share similarities that are much greater than our differences—we all will die and experience loss and most of us will live long enough to have a chronic illness.

The many ways we can find solace by helping each other is at the core of our stories.

Dr. Overman and I believe help is available for your body, mind, and spirit. We believe humor is a great way to cope with what ails you. We believe you are still a citizen of your community and have positive contributions to make, even if that might seem impossible right now. Most importantly, we believe there are phases to living with chronic illness and each phase has its own set of challenges, opportunities, and lessons. By helping to guide you through these phases we believe you will discover that your future, even with a chronic illness, does not have to be dismal, rather you can build a future that is peaceful and rich with meaning.

You will find many stories in the pages to come, written by both Dr. Overman and myself. This is because we believe the important things in life are most vividly expressed in stories and stories are a great teacher, much better than a lot of advice and rules for you to follow. We hope that by sharing our stories about living with and treating chronic illness, you might benefit from our experiences and find in these pages a roadmap that will help you on your own journey.

The story of my own strange symptoms first began in the 1980s when I was in my late 30s. Like many chronic illnesses, mine began with vague, but steadily worsening, symptoms of pain, fatigue, sleeplessness, and memory loss. As time went on, I experienced allergies and asthma, bowel and bladder disorders, and skin irritations. The pain, which began in my pelvis, became worse and generalized. It seemed as if my body was at war with itself and my environment.

I reported these symptoms to various doctors over seven years before I received my first diagnosis. It took another three years of searching before I assembled a team of doctors, led by rheumatologist Dr. Steve Overman, with whom I could communicate and build trust. Slowly, and with my doctors' help, I gained the tools to manage my symptoms, accepted that my illness was chronic, and made peace with the quiet lifestyle that illness demands. I was shattered with grief at the loss of the person I once was, but in time I built a new life and no longer felt regret at the turn my life had taken. Without realizing it at the time,

I had passed through what Dr. Overman and I came to call the Four Phases of Invisible Chronic Illness. They are:

- Getting Sick
- Being Sick
- Grief and Acceptance
- Living Well

My first seven years of searching for answers is what we call the difficult *Getting Sick* phase. As I learned to understand and better manage my symptoms and gain control over the health care I received, I passed through the *Being Sick* phase. Over and over again, I experienced the third phase *Grief* at the loss of the person I used to be, followed by *Acceptance* of the person I had become. This grief was deepest when I confronted the reality that my illness was not going to go away. Eventually, as I made peace with my new circumstances, I found the path to *Living Well* and began to enjoy my new life—a life that contained long-term illness.

DR. OVERMAN

Joy and I had already spent some time talking about Joy's three stages of illness when I heard Patricia Fennell, MSW, LCSW-R, speak about her own research on chronic illness. It gave credence to Joy's experience that Fennell also divided chronic illness into phases. In 1993, she began publishing data on the Fennell Four Phase Model, comprised of Crisis, Stabilization, Resolution, and Integration.™ The Four Phase Model is discussed extensively in her books and articles, including *Managing Chronic Illness Using the Four-Phase Approach, The Chronic Illness Workbook* (2001, 2012), and the *Handbook of Chronic Fatigue Syndrome and Fatiguing Illnesses (2003)(1)*.

In the first edition of our book we divided Joy's illness into three stages *(Getting Sick, Being Sick, and Living Well)*. Joy wrote extensively throughout about her grief at the loss of function and her work identity and how she had to come to terms with this loss to begin to build a new life. After publication, we continued to work with these ideas in Joy's life and in my practice. We came to see that although grief can recur over and over throughout the illness journey, it is a necessary phase that must be navigated in order to begin to live well with illness. So in this edition, we add *Grief and Acceptance* as a defined third of four phases and have grouped our stories accordingly.

Joy's experience can be described to reflect Fennell's Four Phase Model. Fennell's first phase, *Crisis*, includes the anger, fear, and loss, which Joy experienced while getting sick. In Fennell's second phase, *Stabilization*, Joy tells stories of being sick and putting into action a plan for managing her illness and her life. Joy's grief and acceptance of illness as a part of her life is Fennell's third phase, *Resolution*. Finally, Joy began living well as she found value, meaning, and purpose in her new life during her fourth phase, Fennell's *Integration* phase.

In working with my patients, I have observed that learning to live well with illness is not like reaching a destination. They frequently experience repeated episodes of fear, anger, and loss. It is a difficult challenge to accept that no matter how well they manage their illness, their symptoms are now part of their lives and their identity. Even if patients make positive lifestyle changes, and medical advances and new treatments result in regained good health, the experience of chronic illness will still have been life altering. Joy's journey demonstrates how even an experience as devastating as illness can be used by each of us to learn, grow, and become a different, and better, person.

JOY

Coming to terms with my new reality was similar to accepting the death of a loved one. The life I had was gone and I had to bury it, grieve, and go on. Sometimes, on a bad day, I remember my old self, and how my life used to be, and I grow sad. Most of the time, however, I love my life the way it is now, good days and bad. Very early in my illness, my husband and I moved to a small island in the Pacific Northwest, and illness afforded me time to be still and truly see the wondrous beauty of this unique place. Later we moved to my home state of Texas, and I felt the deep emotional connection I had as a child to this land and its hospitable people. Through my struggles, I've learned to live more in the present moment and appreciate any small blessings that may come along each day. Illness made me a better person. I am not so quick to judge people and their actions, now that I know what it feels like to be judged unfairly. Illness has also given me the time to pursue quiet interests that were once stored away in the attic of my life, waiting for a rainy day. I am no longer sorry that the long, rainy day came for me.

Like millions of people who become chronically ill in their prime, but do not die prematurely, I have also had to face the fact that I am likely to live more than half my life ill. It only makes practical sense for me to use this precious time to fashion a fulfilling life, one that includes my illness.

DR. OVERMAN

There have been significant changes in the national conversation around health care since we published the first edition of *You Don't LOOK Sick*. Congress passed the Affordable Health Care Act in 2010, but the debate goes on. We have all heard chronic illness care addressed during this debate, usually in terms of how much it costs to treat and care for chronically ill patients. The debate rarely considers the patient perspective, nor does it focus on how poorly we, as a nation, meet patient needs. I feel that our nation needs to hear stories like Joy's, and yours, about the realities of living with chronic illness.

Let me offer some basic definitions about chronic illness so that we have a shared understanding of the terms. By general definition, a chronic condition lasts more than three months and most have the following general characteristics in common:

- The illness is treatable, but the cure is unknown.
- The causes are often unknown or poorly understood.
- Related symptoms are persistent and recurring.
- Remissions are possible, but unpredictable, and often temporary.

Don't let this definition cause you to lose hope; we are making progress. Although many chronic illnesses have no known cause, others now have a partial answer such as the insulin deficiency in diabetes. We are learning more every day about genetic and environmental factors that can cause chronic disease. For example, certain genes, such as the *HLA DQ2* or *DQ8*, are almost always present in persons with celiac disease. While we have long known that smoking is a risk factor in cancer, we now know it also increases the risk of rheumatoid arthritis.

By contrast, an *acute* illness has a quick or serious onset of symptoms and a more clearly defined prognosis. A person with an acute illness generally gets sick and, in short order, is either cured or dies. With successful treatment, some acute illnesses can develop into chronic illnesses. For example, with advances in treatment, many forms of cancer and human immunodeficiency virus (HIV)-related illnesses that were once terminal have now evolved into manageable chronic illnesses. Understanding how an acute illness affects the immune, metabolic, nervous, and transport systems is also critical to understanding why so many different chronic illnesses have symptoms in common, such as pain, fatigue, sleep disorders, changes in weight, poor function, susceptibility to infection, dietary sensitivities, and emotional irritability.

JOY

During the seven long years I spent searching for answers before I received my first diagnosis, my physicians sometimes got inconclusive results on their medical tests and consequently were either dismissive of my symptoms or minimized them. It was up to me to keep looking. Even after I was diagnosed with a bladder disease, interstitial cystitis, and began to receive treatment, I knew the search was not over as there was more going on with me than just this illness. When I found my way to Dr. Overman, I learned I also had an autoimmune disease: undifferentiated connective tissue disease. This meant my immune system was out of balance and attacking me instead of helping me to heal. The label *undifferentiated* meant I had symptoms common to many autoimmune disorders, but did not test as classic for any particular one.

Other doctors added the diagnosis of fibromyalgia, a disorder of amplified, widespread pain. Putting a name to what was wrong not only gave me resolution and the opportunity for effective treatment, but allowed me to put aside the deep fear that I was going to die from my ailments.

Later, the national press began to report on women becoming ill from silicone breast implants. I had implants and decided to have surgery to remove them. If there was any chance they might be making me ill, I wanted to take action. During the surgery, my doctor found one of the implants had ruptured and the silicone gel had leaked into my body. Now, I had a whole new and poorly understood complication to add to my mix of symptoms and the possible causes.

A few years after that, I began to have pain along the upper jaw line on the right side of my face. Once again, I spent three years searching for the cause, with the pain continually worsening. I underwent many dental procedures and even sinus surgery before I finally learned I had a neurological disorder called trigeminal neuralgia, also a chronic condition. It could be treated with medication, but I was offered no hope for a cure at that time. I was thrust once again into the phase of *Being Sick* as I worked with my doctor to find the best treatment and altered my lifestyle to manage my symptoms. I also experienced another phase of *Grief and Acceptance*.

At first this new diagnosis, which seemed so unrelated to the others, really took me to my knees and seemed to be more than I could bear. Did I really have to endure *another* painful chronic condition? It was tempting to descend into self-pity, but I was more experienced at working my way through these feelings and able to move through this phase with more skill and ease.

I am grateful this journey gets easier with time, but it is still hard to understand why just identifying what was wrong with me took so many years. From speaking to other patients around the country, I know that my story is not unusual.

DR. OVERMAN

Arthritis, musculoskeletal pain, and neuromuscular and auto-immune disorders represent *the most common causes* of disability due to illness in the United States today. These include illnesses such as rheumatoid arthritis, osteoarthritis, Sjögren's syndrome, lupus, Crohn's disease, degenerative disc disease, fibromyalgia, chronic fatigue syndrome, celiac disease, multiple sclerosis, Hashimoto's thyroiditis, spondylitis, and even chronic low back pain. Although each condition has its own unique features, they also have similar symptoms that can be disabling to patients, such as muscle and joint pain, nerve pain, chronic fatigue, sleep disturbance, short-term memory loss, skin sensitivity, bowel or bladder abnormalities, allergies, and sometimes organ involvement. Tens of millions of people have these illnesses and each year they spend billions of dollars seeking effective treatment. It should not take Joy, or anyone else, multiple years to get a diagnosis. I understand the frustration.

My specialty, rheumatology, is focused on the diagnosis and treatment of complex, chronic illnesses like the ones I have described above, but the primary focus of modern Western medicine has been to identify acute illnesses and treat them with acute interventions, such as surgery or antibiotics. Although Western doctors can take justifiable pride in our advanced abilities to offer the high-tech quick fix, our system has yet to catch up with other countries in meeting the needs of persons with chronic conditions, a group whose numbers are growing as our life span increases. The focus of our medical education, research investment, and insurance compensation also fail to meet the increasing needs of the chronically ill. Too many physicians lack the skill, and sometimes the interest, to offer diagnosis and ongoing care for the chronically ill, especially those with chronic pain syndromes.

Chronic illness care requires a lot of time—time to listen to the story, assess the physiology of the conditions, evaluate the risks and benefits of various medications, and help patients understand the expected phases of their illness. Because all this is so time consuming, it frequently leads our overworked and poorly equipped primary care physicians to treat symptoms only, without diagnosing and addressing the underlying medical, environmental, or lifestyle causes of the illness. In other words, they find themselves unable to care for the whole person. Unfortunately, our insurance system pays highly for procedures like surgery, laboratory tests, and diagnostic radiology, but much less for the time spent in communication with patients. The arbitrary way these payment priorities are set has resulted in fewer physicians entering chronic illness care specialties. Patients in need find they are often limited to only fifteen-minute visits with their physician.

An understanding of the label *syndrome* will further illustrate the difficulty in making a clear diagnosis. A syndrome is simply a poorly understood illness. It is often initially defined for research purposes and given a name because sufficient laboratory, clinical, or symptom criteria are present. A syndrome may have more than one cause and symptoms that are not unique to it. The label *syndrome* does not mean the illness is not real, but rather that the medical community still does not understand it well enough to call it a disease.

For example, Joy's fibromyalgia is a chronic pain syndrome and was until recently diagnosed by a patient reporting pain that occurs with pressure on eleven out of eighteen specific points around the body. Now, in an effort to better understand the illness, there are recommendations to drop the examination findings of tenderness from the diagnosis of fibromyalgia, and instead use only symptom criteria. This is partially because tenderness at these points can frequently be attributed to other causes, such as tennis elbow or neck strain. We also know now that fibromyalgia patients usually have a variety of symptoms beyond those of musculoskeletal pain and tenderness. For example, as was true in Joy's case, patients often report nonrestorative sleep, irritable bowel symptoms, bladder urgency, cognitive problems, anxiety, and fatigue. Fibromyalgia is now thought to be a syndrome of nervous system amplification. This means the nervous system is more sensitive to all stimuli and therefore magnifies the reporting to your brain. Light touch may feel like pain and normal bodily sensations may be uncomfortable.

Many women with fibromyalgia are also diagnosed with chronic fatigue syndrome, or CFS. But can you have two syndromes, or more, at once? The answer is yes, but CFS has different diagnosis requirements than fibromyalgia. CFS is a diagnosis of exclusion, meaning that other causes of fatigue must be ruled out. Fibromyalgia can be inclusive. For example, if you have rheumatoid arthritis or lupus, and you also have the tenderness of a sensitized nervous system, you can meet the criteria for fibromyalgia.

I usually tell new patients that getting the diagnosis of fibromyalgia is like being told that those dark spots on your body are bruises. Immediately you would ask the question most important to you—what is causing the bruises? With fibromyalgia, the diagnosis is only the beginning of the search for answers. Next we must ask, is your illness caused or triggered by inflammatory illness, sleep disorder, stress, metabolic problems, or neck injury? While the medical literature does not clarify these distinctions, I tell my patients that it takes problems in at least two of these domains to disrupt the balance of the nervous system to a degree that leads to the widespread body sensitivity called fibromyalgia.

Chronic fatigue syndrome is different. CFS has specific diagnostic criteria a patient must have:

- Clinically evaluated, unexplained, persistent, or relapsing fatigue that is of new or definite onset.
- Not the result of ongoing exertion.
- Not alleviated by rest.
- Results in substantial reduction in previous levels of occupational, educational, social, or personal activities.

In addition, patients need to have four or more of the following symptoms that persist or recur during six or more consecutive months of illness and that do not predate the fatigue: self-reported impairment in short-term memory or concentration, sore throat, tender cervical or axillary nodes, muscle pain, multi-joint pain without redness or swelling, headaches of a new pattern or severity, sleep that is not refreshing, or post-exertion malaise lasting longer than 24 hours. Note that the word *unexplained* means other causes have been ruled out, with the exception of fibromyalgia, since it occurs so frequently with CFS. So if you are beginning to think this whole process of figuring out what is wrong, what caused it, and what to do about it is extremely complicated, you can imagine how a primary care physician feels when asked to assess and effectively treat a patient reporting these symptoms.

Fatigue is one of the most common symptoms reported to primary care physicians, occurring in a quarter of the individuals who enter their offices, and it is more commonly reported by women than by men. Epidemiology researchers make the CFS syndrome definition restrictive so as to exclude common, known causes of fatigue. This strategy maximizes the chances that research studies will detect significant associations with a specific cause or group of factors that lead to CFS. Though this clinical case definition is well established, its strict use may not always be appropriate in the evaluation of a specific patient. For me, these strict criteria are useful as a constant reminder that there are many diseases or other syndromes that may present like CFS or just fatigue in general. Since there is no known treatment for persons with classic CFS, I rarely put the label CFS on my problem list for a patient. Instead, I usually list the various symptoms that are present so that I am constantly looking for patterns that might lead to other diagnoses that are known to be treatable. Yes, this is complicated and it is why rheumatology is both an exciting and challenging specialty, and why I have gray hair!

Even though we don't fully understand how or why, I believe all of Joy's diagnoses are likely related to one another, much like the elephant that was really one beast, even though each of the blind examiners could only identify the separate parts.

JOY

It wouldn't make much difference if the blind men could see all of me, since so few of my symptoms are visible. Since I don't look sick, I don't get much acknowledgment for being sick either. Often people are downright skeptical about the reality of my illnesses, and say so. I wasn't able to find many books to prepare me for the real world of living with illnesses like mine. Most of the books in the health section promised to explain "Everything You Ever Wanted to Know" about one specific disease. I have more than one illness, with symptoms that overlap, so this perspective was of limited help. I found other books that offered the "Seven Easy Steps to the Cure." I thought these books implied that if the promised cure didn't happen for me, it was somehow my own fault. If my well-trained doctors could not offer me a cure for my illnesses, the last thing I needed to do was blame myself for failing to do so.

I decided I should write the book I could not find, but wanted to read. It wouldn't overwhelm the reader with technical information or promise an easy fix, but it would make them feel *recognized*. Readers would know they weren't alone in feeling scared and angry. They would feel empowered to fight for their rights and needs. I could offer hope that finding peace and personal growth can be a part of the long-term illness experience. If I could share my stories about the physical and emotional phases I went through in dealing with the impact of multiple chronic illnesses, and how I traveled through these phases, maybe I could help others get started on their way.

I asked Dr. Overman if he would write the book with me. It took me a long time to find Dr. Overman, and I thought by demonstrating how we work together, readers would be encouraged to keep looking until they found the right doctor for them. He could add his professional insight and wisdom and share other patients' stories, so readers would get more than just my experience. Between the two of us, perhaps the book could become a useful road map to guide others on a journey to a better life with illness.

DR. OVERMAN

When Joy first asked me to write a book with her, I casually said, "Sure," assuming the idea would pass. Obviously, I didn't know Joy very well yet, but I was curious and began to talk to my patients about these ideas. I asked, "What would be your best advice to help someone live well with a chronic illness?"

One patient, Sharon, gave my question some thought, and then wrote this insightful response: "To live well, you need to understand that in a fast-paced, success-oriented society you are still valuable, even though you may be bedridden, unemployed, or suffering from chronic pain. The way to do this is to retain a positive self-image and a sense of usefulness. This is difficult to do, but essential."

The next time Joy asked me to co-author her book, I realized she was serious and I was hooked. I responded with a sincere and enthusiastic, "Yes!"

JOY

Working with Dr. Overman as my physician, teacher, co-author, and friend has really helped me cope with my illness in a positive way. I've had other advantages, too. I have a large and supportive family and my children were grown and on their own before I became seriously ill. I had a professional career that gave me confidence in dealing with other professionals, like physicians. Through my employer, I had excellent medical and disability insurance. I went on long-term disability in 1994 and my contract enabled me to continue to receive an income that made me feel safe.

I had worked in finance and knew something about corporations and the importance of corporate earnings, so when I had to deal with insurance companies and their denied claims, impersonal treatment, and logjams of paperwork, it made me mad but I realized it wasn't really about me. They were merely applying what they call risk management. After I became sick, they were spending more money to cover my claims than they were receiving in premiums. Though I had been a profitable client for these companies for many years, this current imbalance was a threat to their bottom line and to shareholder value. One result of having a for-profit, and often publicly traded, health insurance system in America is that corporations may be motivated to make decisions that benefit business goals more than public health care needs. This fact puts patient needs further down the pipeline than they should be. For example, people like me who work for large corporations often enjoy better insurance packages because large corporations can negotiate more favorable insurance rates than a small employer or the self-employed. Those of us who are seriously ill collectively bear the consequences resulting from this discrimination and conflict of interest, and it is our job to fight for all patients' rights and needs.

The security I am fortunate enough to enjoy in my life gave me the time and freedom to take on the big task of writing this book. Those of you who read it might not be as secure, and therefore have an even more difficult journey than mine. Please know that I sympathize with you and will continue to do all I can to advocate for you and improve the system to better serve the needs of those with chronic illness.

DR. OVERMAN

Unfortunately, what Joy experienced with her insurers is too often the norm, and our health care system continues to provide inadequate care for the millions of people with chronic conditions. However, even as positive change occurs, learning to live well with an invisible chronic illness will remain a challenging, personal journey. To help you meet the challenge, we share three of Joy's stories we believe are common to many in each phase of the illness. These are followed by my own stories, professional insights, and tips to support your successful progress through this phase. At the end of the book we offer online resources and names of patient support organizations, as well as discussion questions, to promote your deepening knowledge.

Each of you will have your own unique journey to take, teenagers to octogenarians, men as well as women, singly or with a partner, and the life experiences that allow you to grow and come to terms with illness will surely be different than ours. It is our hope that as you read our stories, you will be prompted to consider the ways your own experiences might offer opportunities to better understand your chronic illness. We hope our book helps you find your way from *Getting Sick* to *Being Sick* and to navigate your *Grief* and find *Acceptance* in your new life. Joy and I both wish you well in your journey all the way to *Living Well.*

Phase I
Getting Sick

Snake in the Mist

The Seattle porch where I sit this fall night is wet and shrouded in a chilling fog. I can't see two feet in front of me. I try to push aside the curtain of mist to peer through it, but my hand moves as if through water, the moisture quickly backfilling the slight cavity I have made. I am afraid of this dense dark, and I am dismayed that I am powerless to penetrate it even slightly. I fear there may be something out there I can't see, like a snake in the mist, poised and waiting to strike me.

The truth is I am just afraid. I have come to Seattle for a medical test, one of a series of medical tests that only seem to raise questions without offering answers. Before this one today, there have been many other days of many other tests, resulting in no more than guesses and stabs at naming all that is wrong with me. I believe I have done the best I can to help find the answers. I have gone to dozens of doctors, read volumes of research, and sought the advice of alternative health care practitioners. Yet I am still so lost, so confused, and so frightened. I am still so very, very ill.

After the test today, I am tired and hurting. I will stay tonight in Seattle with dear friends. They, sensing my despair, gave me dinner and hugs and wished me well, and then wisely left me alone with my thoughts, here on their dank porch.

I reflect that it has been seven years since I first sensed that something was wrong with me and began reporting symptoms to my doctors. It has been over a year since I began a determined search to finally find out just what it is and what to do about it. I wonder if I have moved from the spot where I first began. I need someone to lead me, a good doctor in whom I can place my trust. Should that be so hard to find? Yes, my experience tells me, yes, it is just as hard to find a partner in illness as it is to find a partner in life.

That is not to say I haven't been able to find any good doctors, I have. But I don't have that one special doctor. I have had a hysterectomy at the recommendation of a respected gynecologist. I think he did a good job, but his surgery did not make me well. I went to see a neurologist who, gratefully, has ruled out that I have multiple sclerosis, which might have explained my clumsiness, my inability to think straight, and my fatigue. He has referred me to a rheumatologist who is treating women made sick from silicone breast implants. Perhaps this doctor will find my symptoms familiar and will have some experience in how to treat them. So far, none of my efforts, or these doctors' efforts, have improved my health, or even clearly explained what is making me so sick.

Today's tests were an attempt to identify the cause of sudden, acute episodes of pelvic pain I have had since the hysterectomy. The first time it happened the pain was so severe, and escalated so intensely, my local island doctor had me flown to the nearest hospital, fearing kidney stones or appendicitis, but it was neither. Then it happened again, and again. Today's ultrasound was inconclusive, but the technician said my left ovary is a little enlarged. When I asked what could cause that swelling, she said, among other possibilities, ovarian cancer. She did not think it was cancer, but in my fearsome state that was all I really heard her say—cancer. Ovarian cancer. A killer cancer.

Now, sitting on this porch in the dark and the wet, I still hear her words ringing in my ears, clanging around in my head, and I know this is the source of my fear—that I will die. I-am-afraid-I-am-going-to-die. I am afraid I am going to die before I even find out what is killing me.

Again, I reach out my hand to try to part the mist, and again I cannot penetrate it. I cannot see a thing out there, but I fear that what I can't see is coming right at me. The death sentence. The snake in the mist.

Three Strikes

A fter waiting in the lobby for forty minutes, I am now sitting in a child-sized chair in the office of a bow-tied and bespectacled urologist. He is sitting in a grown-up chair behind his grown-up desk, ignoring me while reviewing my file. This is only our third meeting, but I doubt that I will back for a fourth. I adhere to a "Three Strikes" policy and once I've called the third strike on a doctor, I move on. At our first meeting, this doctor kept me waiting forty-five minutes, and another thirty-five minutes for the second, so I've already called Strike One. I was offered no apology for this, even though common courtesy would dictate that my time is as valuable as his. Besides, if he can't even manage his own schedule, how good can he be at managing my illness?

He has given me my first actual diagnosis, though, which is a relief. He says I have a chronic bladder disease with a wicked-sounding name—interstitial cystitis. He has prescribed for me the medication most commonly used in its treatment, which I am mortified to learn is the same medication given to young children who wet the bed. He has also offered his opinion that there is clearly something else going on with me, yet to be diagnosed, as my set of symptoms are not "classic" for interstitial cystitis. Today I am here to discuss my progress.

"Since I started on the medication, I've been having a rapid, irregular heartbeat," I tell him.

"All the time?" He pops the top off his old-fashioned fountain pen.

"No, mostly in the morning, and mostly at rest."

"That's an unusual side effect."

"It's listed on the package literature, I checked," I say, feeling I have to justify my report.

"Well," he peers at me suspiciously over his glasses, "none of my other patients has ever reported that side effect."

Strike Two! It's not my job to be like his other patients.

I move the meeting along to my next concern. "I had a surgery once and they found a big adhesion right on my bladder. Do you think that could have been a factor in causing this disease?"

"Absolutely not," he answers smugly. "The outside of the bladder is entirely separate from the inside of the bladder. No relationship." He relaxes in his chair, back in control.

"I guess that means you're not a big fan of holistic medicine then, where everything is pretty much assumed to be related to everything else."

He snorts.

"Okay, let me ask you this—you know this big controversy over the safety of silicone breast implants?"

A second snort answers that question.

"I have implants and I've read that a lot of the sick silicone women also have bladder dysfunction."

"Well, I know all about that lawsuit against breast implants, young lady, and I can tell you it's about one thing, and one thing only—lawyers making money. There's no science to it. It's a big bunch of hooey. Besides," he attests, "I have hundreds of male patients with silicone *penile* implants and none of them are sick."

"Really? How do you know?"

"How do I know what?"

"How do you know that silicone didn't make any of your male implant patients sick?"

"What do you mean, how do I know?"

"Well, who are they, a bunch of old guys?"

"Mature."

"Okay, mature. Do any of them ever report debilitating fatigue or memory loss?"

"Certainly."

"How about joint and muscle pain?"

"Of course."

"Why do you say, of course?"

"Because they're old."

"Mature," I remind him. "Anyway, aren't those the same symptoms the lawsuit claims the women are reporting?"

"I suppose so. I never thought about it."

"So, if you did think about it, isn't it possible your male implant patients could also be having a reaction to silicone? I mean, have you given them tests or anything? How do you know for sure?"

"Because..." he pauses, lowers his chin, takes a bead on me over the tops of his glasses, and repeats, "Because, young lady, I'm the doctor. That's how I know."

STEE-RIKE THU-REE! I am out of here!

I struggle out of my little chair, hoist my big-girl briefcase onto my shoulder, and thrust out my hand to him. In the most polite voice I can muster I say, "Thank you for your time today. I think I will take a break from that medication for a little while. You know, give my heart rate a chance to calm down."

He shrugs, offers me a limp handshake and I leave.

I will not be back. It's not that this urologist is a bad person, or necessarily even a bad doctor. To be fair, I did confront him on an issue that was not in his area of expertise. Still, he talked down to me as if I were a child, a lesser person. I need to find a doctor who will treat me like a grown up, thinking person, not act like a scolding parent. I want a doctor who can become my health care partner, and I don't think this man would ever be willing to do that. In order for the partnership I envision to work, there are certain things we would both need to commit to do:

- We must treat each other with courtesy.
- We must see each other as unique.
- We must be as honest and informed as we possibly can.
- We must be willing to work together to build trust.

7

I am willing to do this, and I don't think that it is too much to ask of my doctor. This relationship is too important to settle for less, so I'll just have to keep on looking. I know there is a doctor out there somewhere, just right for me.

Pills, Procedures, and Paperwork

The good news is I have two great doctors and three actual, treatable diagnoses now: interstitial cystitis, mixed connective tissue disease, and fibromyalgia. The not so good news is I feel like a lab rat. I've been pricked and poked and prodded and photographed more times in the last year than in all my previous years put together. After my first urologist struck out, I started asking around for a referral, a doctor who really knew something about interstitial cystitis. Often I can get the best referrals from practicing nurses, but this time it came from a physician I met at a garden party. He told me I could find a leading female doctor in this field at the University of Washington Medical School in Seattle. I called for an appointment the very next day and found my perfect fit. She is eager, interested, and has lots of patients with a diagnosis of interstitial cystitis.

I also started asking around for the name of a physician treating women who have become ill from silicone breast implants. I don't know if this is what is wrong with me, but there is so much press about it that cite symptoms similar to mine I've become suspicious. Recently when I saw my neurologist, I asked him if he could give me a referral.

"There are only two docs in town treating these women that I know of," he said. "They are rheumatologists and both are at Minor and James."

I wouldn't have thought to look for a rheumatologist, I thought they were doctors for old people, but on this advice I called for an appointment.

Dr. Overman actually took my call personally. "I'm on call this weekend," he said. "I have to be in the office anyway, so why don't you come on in?"

I was sold before I even met him, and once I did he diagnosed and began treating me for mixed connective tissue disease, an autoimmune disorder. MCTD is the label used when a patient exhibits individual symptoms that may be common to several diseases, but taken together are classic for none. He said that many of the women with silicone breast implants who have become ill have this diagnosis. I have the dry mouth and eyes of Sjögren's syndrome, the aching joints of arthritis, the deep fatigue of lupus, but lab tests are inconclusive and don't confirm any of these. He also says I meet the diagnostic criteria for fibromyalgia, yet another mystery disease. Dr. Overman, like my new urologist, believes what I report and is determined to find answers that will improve my function and quality of life, even if he can't offer me a cure. After my long search for just one good doctor, I feel like I have landed in Dr. Nirvana.

Overcome with gratitude, I am determined to be the best patient I can be. I want to be the patient they are glad to see come through the door each month. To this end, I come prepared for each visit with my trusty yellow legal pad. On it I have written my list of current medications, new, changing, or continuing symptoms, my three questions for the meeting, and room at the bottom to take notes. I know my doctors are always pressed for time, so I choose these three questions carefully.

One day in a meeting, I sit beside Dr. Overman. My chair is the same size as his, like we are both grown-ups. I have my yellow legal pad in my lap and I am reading to him from my list. He is busy taking notes for his ever-expanding file on me. After a few minutes, he leans closer to me, peers at my pad, and says, "Is this our meeting?"

"Yes," I answer proudly.

"Then why don't you give it to me?" He takes the pad from my lap and begins to read for himself with interest.

I'm not sure whether to feel robbed or proud, but I adapt. I make a *Dr. Visit* template for my computer and save it in my own ever-expanding file. For each meeting, I fill out the template and bring two copies with me, one for him to use and keep, and one for me. Both of my new doctors are referring me to other practitioners, so I've also prepared a complete medical history that I take to each new doctor. Now, when the nurse hands me the detailed new patient form to fill out, I can just write, "See Attached." These time-saving devices have greatly helped me to improve my attitude about becoming a career lab rat.

I recently visited an immunologist from Bastyr College of Naturopathic Medicine who drew a blood sample to test me for over 350 food sensitivities and allergies. He says if we can identify the substances that cause my immune system to overreact and avoid them, it might allow my condition to calm down. He seems a little disappointed to find I am sensitive to absolutely nothing. He was hoping he could at least get me to stop drinking coffee. The acupuncturist I am seeing tells me these sensitivities may not indicate an allergy so much as a system out of balance. Certain highly reactive foods, like wheat and milk products, are more likely to signal this imbalance than others, but when the system is brought into proper balance these intolerances may disappear. Somehow both of these views, conflicting on the surface, make sense to me now. I'm learning that issues around illness and health that I once thought of as a straight line—get sick, take medicine, get well—now look more like a sphere. Explore, Understand, Adapt.

My medical insurer has suddenly got me on their radar. I think they have put a big red sticker on my file that indicates *Too Many Claims, Not Enough Premiums*. The result is an increase in challenged and denied claims, most recently for chiropractic care. This is serious because my chiropractor is the only practitioner in my small island town who can offer me real relief from a flare of widespread pain. Here's the way I experience it: First, I have a spasm of pelvic pain, originating in my poor, beleaguered bladder. The pain spreads outward and into the nerves that exit my bladder, traveling along this neural highway until it enters my sacrum. I feel as if something reaches out and gives my sacrum a yank, which alerts my spine and the pain travels straight up, vertebra by vertebra, until it reaches my neck. Then the pain control knob in my brain starts to move the dial higher until my entire central nervous system becomes involved and pain fans out to my whole body, into every one of my limbs and penetrates all my tissues. Ultimately, it hurts to press my finger against my skin.

The remedy is to go see the chiropractor. He sets the now swollen sacrum back in place, adjusts my pelvis, does some acupressure on my spine, and the process begins to reverse itself. The pain control knob in the brain turns the volume back down, the neck and spine relax, and my whole body begins to ease as the pain subdues like a receding tide. I feel like I can exhale again.

The letter from the medical insurer denying coverage for this life altering treatment states that it is not "medically necessary." I call them up and ask what the heck that means. I am told that because the chiropractor has been unable to cure me in a reasonable amount of time, his treatment is not medically necessary. This statement is being made to a woman diagnosed with three chronic conditions that no one has been able to cure in any way whatsoever. I decide to appeal. In order to do this, my chiropractor is required to send in his records, called his S.O.A.P. notes, which stands for Subjective Objective Assessment Plan. This sounds like an oxymoron to me, but so be it.

While I wait for the ruling, I continue to make my monthly trips to the mainland to see my ever-growing stable of health care providers. My urologist has referred me to a physical therapist whose specialty is treating pelvic pain or *myalgia*. She uses biofeedback to help her patients become aware of their involuntary pelvic floor muscles and to learn to intentionally relax them when they spasm. As I come to understand that the brain can communicate with and influence a part of the body whose function is described as involuntary, another of my assumptions about the linear relationship between the mind and body is scuttled. I will not describe exactly how the physical therapist works with me as the "yuck" factor is too great, but let me just say a probe is involved. The learning curve is both steep and embarrassing, but the practice helps. Now when I feel pelvic pain coming on, I can get still, locate those muscles in my mind and will them to relax. This is a small miracle to me.

Urology offers endless opportunity for embarrassment. First of all, it's embarrassing to tell people I have a bladder disease—it's embarrassing to even say the word *bladder* in a social situation. I find I am reluctant to tell people I am sick because they will ask what I have and I don't want to say it out loud. This is a socially isolating position, made worse by the fibromyalgia diagnosis. A lot of people don't believe fibromyalgia is real, plus it's called a syndrome, which makes it sound like a mental illness. I don't like to tell people I have that either. Usually, I just say I have undifferentiated connective tissue disease, which no one has ever heard of and is unpronounceable, therefore more credible. I guess the silver lining in all this is that I have three diagnoses to choose from and at least one of them has some social benefits.

The University of Washington is a teaching hospital and because of this, my urologist often asks if medical students can observe the procedures she does with me. Since I am committed to be her very best patient, I always agree. Recently I found myself sitting in a metal chair so rigged up with wires it looked like a torture machine from a science fiction movie. A roomful of doctors, technicians, and medical students crowd into the exam room while the machine fills my bladder, then empties it, fills, then empties again. We are testing *bladder capacity* and we learn that, unlike many patients with interstitial cystitis, I have plenty of it.

No one is really paying any attention to me, as they are glued to the screen charting the results of the test, but as the machine pumps my bladder beyond full, I am taken back to those terrible childhood memories of having to pee so badly I had to sit with my legs crossed. The adults in my life, after spending months teaching me to pee in a toilet and asking me every ten minutes if I had to go, suddenly reversed their course. Whether in a car, store, restaurant, or classroom, when I told an adult that I had to pee, instead of rushing me to the bathroom as they once had, they would now say, "Can't you wait a while longer?" Much of my childhood was spent desperately waiting for adults to allow me to pee.

Now I sit on the torture chair in this crowded room, squirming with increasing discomfort until, suddenly, the awful memory is replaced by the realization of an even more horrible childhood fear. I feel myself actually peeing in the middle of a room full of strangers. For an entire afternoon, these dual horrors are repeated over, and over, and over, without my having any ability to control them. My urologist is so pleased at my bladder capacity. Good for her. I'm thinking I may not volunteer anymore.

When I return home, I open the mail to find my insurance claim appeal for chiropractic care has been denied. Further, the insurer now declares that my chiropractor's S.O.A.P. notes, the ironic subjective/objective ones, are incomplete. I find this odd since four of the employees in the office where I work see this same chiropractor and the notes have never been deemed inadequate to justify their treatment, nor have any of them ever had a claim denied. It seems the doctor is being held to a different standard only in my case. I decide to appeal again. This time, they want him to provide three years of records on my treatment, in spite of the fact that the claims for these three previous years are not in question. It feels like busy work to me. I think it is the increasing volume of my claims that is being resisted, not just this one. He's just taking the hit. I am lucky he is supportive of me and willing to take up staff time to collect these data.

All these pills, procedures, and paperwork wear me out. Fatigue is an overwhelming struggle, especially since I have to travel to the mainland for care. I find I cannot make the trip in a day, nor can my husband drive me because he must cover my clients in the office where we both work. After I travel an hour and a half on the ferry bound for the mainland, I must drive for another hour and a half to Seattle, with several requisite stops to pee along the way. I have identified the cleanest bathrooms in gas station and fast food restaurants in western Washington. I could write a *User's Guide to the Best Bathrooms*. Once I make it to Seattle, I see a doctor or two in the afternoon, then collapse overnight in a hotel, get up early, and see another one or two in the morning before driving home. I have learned to keep a pillow and comforter in the back seat of my car so I can lie down and rest while I wait in the ferry line for the boat to arrive. I'm often awakened by the sound of the cars behind me honking for me to board. I struggle out of the back, dive into the front seat, drive onto the ferry, return to the back seat, and fall asleep again. Repeat, repeat, repeat.

The second appeal is denied. The insurer writes:

> *After review of the medical documentation submitted, the professional consultant reports to the plan that care is considered chronic/supportive care. There is not objective documentation submitted that verifies the medical necessity of continuing services. The duration of care is not reasonable and customary for the diagnosis on file.*

This reads like a form letter, or a few form letters pieced together. I don't think they are responding to my unique case at all. Besides, all my doctors are offering me chronic/supportive care; most of them just do it with prescription drugs rather than a chiropractic adjustment. I've been to dozens of doctors in the last few years, and filed many dozens of prescription drug claims, but never once has my insurance company questioned the medical necessity of a pill, or required the prescription to be accompanied by objective documentation. I'd speculate a for-profit, corporate health care system sees more opportunity for growing profits in big pharma than among chiropractors.

The insurer allows a final chance to appeal. For this third round, all treating physicians are required to send letters recommending that I continue therapy with the chiropractor. Clever tactic, as they know MDs aren't always entirely supportive of chiropractic care, some even see it as quackery. But mine are willing. They know I am doing many things to help improve my symptoms and this is relief I can get without leaving the island. They trust me when I report that it helps. My urologist, rheumatologist, physical therapist, and chiropractor all provide me with a letter plus their diagnosis and treatment notes for the past three years. All state that this treatment relieves my symptoms and improves my function and quality of life. They acknowledge that with a chronic condition, they can do no more for me themselves. Dr. Overman, as my principal physician, requests that the insurer contact him personally if they intend to deny this claim again. He tells me that when you ask someone way out in insurance land

15

to take the time to talk to a doctor in the real world, they usually just pay the claim. The time it takes to make the call is not worth the money. Ah, that human touch.

Dr. Overman and I continue our efforts at unraveling the complicated mystery of what ails me. My illnesses are poorly understood, which makes treatment a murky stew of possibilities. He tells me the big challenge in treating a case like mine is determining the driver of my chronic pain. Is it inflammation, low serotonin in the brain, the central nervous system? He says treatment itself will teach us. If we choose the right medication, I will get better. If not, I won't. I realize this is contrary to conventional wisdom. I thought that based on the diagnosis, a doctor should be able to choose the right medicine and, bull's-eye, problem solved. But when illnesses are defined with descriptive words like "chronic," "hard to diagnose," "difficult to treat," and "poorly understood" as mine are, this protocol is reversed. Further, Dr. Overman tells me, it's not just one medication that we seek; rather, we will likely end up with several medications in a subtle variety of doses and add to that any alternative therapies that might help. He says that even when we do find a combination that works, we must continue to monitor my response because it is likely to change over time. The protocol will need to be adjusted as I get better, new symptoms arise, or my tolerance for the medication changes. In order to be an effective partner, I must learn to pay close attention to my symptoms so I can report them accurately. I have to learn a new language to describe what I am feeling and experiencing so that it is clear to him, and then he can help me. This same process is going on with all my prescribing physicians; I find the demands endless and exhausting.

At the end of the year, to try to bring order to this confusion and overlap, I decide to provide my physicians with an Annual Report. I need to do this for myself to sort it all out, so I reason that they might find it helpful, too. I write a brief history of the year, including all the treatments I've tried and the outcomes I've experienced. I outline the symptoms at year end and the medications I am currently taking. I list the names and specialties of my treating physicians and their contact information, and I send a copy of the report to each one of them. They like it, I get a gold star. If there was a Patient of the Year award, I might have a shot. Now when I go to an appointment, I often find my doctor at the desk reviewing my Annual Report in preparation for our meeting.

My medical insurer does not contact Dr. Overman about my appeal as requested and, again, the claim is denied. I am told there are no more appeals allowed; the case is closed. I review my contract with the insurer. It says I am entitled to up to 20 chiropractic visits annually. They denied coverage of my treatment in September, after only 15 visits. I decide to contact my employer. My company signed a contract with this insurer on behalf of all their employees and is paying a lot for the service. I want to see if the way I am being treated meets their expectations. The insurer may be in the business of collecting premiums and denying claims, but I bet my employer is in the business of getting their money's worth. I send the entire file to Human Resources including a cover letter that tracks the appeal process. I write that all I want is coverage for the 20 visits annually outlined in my contract and I would expect to pay out of pocket after that. If this denial of claim does not match the expectations my employer had when they hired this insurer, I ask that they intervene on my behalf.

A month and a half later, I receive a check for $665.60 in the mail, reimbursement for the 9 months of denied claims that I've submitted during this process. This time the cover letter has only this brief statement:

> *Remark code 22: We have reconsidered these charges because of additional information we received.*

I bet they got some additional information! I guess it's true what they say—it's the squeaky wheel that gets the grease and $665 is a lot of grease. I send a thank you note to the head of my employer's Human Resources Department.

This journey through pills, procedures, and paperwork is teaching me something. I had thought of illness as something that happened *to* me, like an attack from an unseen enemy—that snake in the mist. My work with my physicians is teaching me that this illness *is* me. Not all of me, but a big part of me. I'm learning that what I must think of as *me* includes the mind, the body, and the spirit all together and this union is a lot more complicated and interdependent than I realized. I am reminded of all my years studying ballet and how I was taught to perform through injury and pain, to use my mind to deny the body. Although this denial is at the core of the grueling discipline of classical ballet, I realize now I must unlearn that skill. Instead, I need to listen to my body and respect my limitations. I need to live within them. I'm just at the beginning of where this experience might take me, but I am learning and I am changing. I am no longer just *getting* sick; I am learning how to *be* sick—the best I can.

Dr. Overman on Getting Sick: The Stuck Car

Most patients come to see a rheumatologist only after seeing many other doctors. They have had many tests. They are often tired, scared, frustrated, and in pain. Their trust in physicians is low and their hope that they will find answers diminished. They know stress makes them feel worse, but since they don't understand what is wrong and why they got sick in the first place, they are confused and understandably stressed. Does this sound like you now? To help, I need to start by listening to your story. Your story is the most important data for making proper diagnoses. If I learn from your story that you are in the *Getting Sick* phase, I might ask, "Do you feel stuck?"

If your answer is yes, I offer this analogy. Let's say you've been driving down the road in your car enjoying the scenery, when suddenly you hit a bump, swerve, go off the road, and find yourself stuck in a muddy ditch. You push on the accelerator, but instead of the car moving forward, your tires spin. You try again, pushing harder on the accelerator, but the tires whirl and your car digs down even deeper. You don't understand why you can't get out of the ditch; you are doing what has worked for you in the past. Then you hear an awful new whine. This noise worries you, but you are not aware that pushing on the accelerator is causing it.

The tires spinning, the wheels digging deeper, and the whining noise as the engine begins to overheat are all mounting warning signs. You might hear these sounds, but maybe you aren't really *listening* to them. *Listening* is a deeper effort and involves trying to understand meanings and looking for patterns or explanations. Why aren't you listening? Perhaps it is because these sounds are brand new to you. Perhaps you are distracted by frustration, or worried about being late. Maybe the only thing you can hear is that voice in your head saying that whatever is going on is all your own fault.

Many new patients come to me after their car has been stuck in the ditch for so long that they feel exhausted and defeated. They fear the worst. They've tried and tried to find answers and get well, with no success. Some have endured months of treatment for the wrong diagnosis. Maybe friends, family, co-workers, or other health care providers have suggested they weren't trying hard enough, their symptoms were all in their head, or they were just depressed. This overwhelming pile up—a lack of experience with illness, worry, frustration, and blame can understandably prevent patients from recognizing they are spinning their wheels and digging themselves deeper and deeper into the ditch.

By the time they get to me, patients often feel defensive and resist any suggestion of mine that anything they are doing might be making their illness worse. I try to reassure them that managing their illness is not only about trying hard. It's about how illness, like that stuck car, is affected by how we deal with it. If patients are unable to communicate effectively with their physician, family, friends, and other providers, the team that might be able to assist them can also become stuck ankle deep in mud, some pushing, others pulling, and everyone out of synch.

There is a complex relationship between the events that cause an illness and factors that perpetuate, or aggravate, it. Returning to the stuck car analogy, there may be pre-existing factors different from those that forced a person into the ditch that will make getting out more difficult. These may be things no one noticed, like thin treads on the tires or a near-empty gas tank. Maybe the oil was low and needed to be changed, or the engine needed a tune up. All these factors, in addition to the event that sent the car off the road in the first place, may be contributing to a patient's difficulty in getting unstuck and back on the road again.

So how might I help you? I am not a tow truck, after all. First, I can throw sand under the tires by diagnosing and treating problems. I can call for help by coordinating an integrated care program and communicating with your family, friends, and other clinicians on your behalf. Perhaps we need to add oil, its absence having caused the engine to overheat, similar to how low brain serotonin levels may lead to inflammation, anxiety, or depression. I can teach you how to listen to what your car is telling you through mind and body awareness, and relaxation and movement therapy.

I must help you take one more essential step. You must learn to drive differently. A chronic illness requires that you accelerate slowly, feel for traction, and ease off the gas pedal if your tires start to spin. You must realize that proper maintenance and repairs take a finely tuned team. Maybe you've reached the point where you feel you have tried everything and now you want it all to be up to me. Just *figure it out* and *fix it*! Sorry, I cannot drive for you or pull you out of the ditch all by myself. I am willing to be your team captain, but I cannot do for you what you must learn to do for yourself, and I am only one committed member of the team you need to put in place.

This first phase, *Getting Sick*, is about crisis—the crisis of not knowing what is happening to you, not having a doctor you can trust, not being able to find a diagnosis [1]. People are unique; they may have defined injures or triggering events, or they have been on a slow slide into sickness, but what they all have in common at this stage is *fear*. What they are missing is *hope*. Creating hope is my job, so here are some Travel Tips that might help you, like Joy, find that hope and move out of the frightening crisis phase of Getting Sick.

FREE YOURSELF FROM THE PRISON OF FEAR

In this first phase, *Getting Sick*, Joy goes through many emotional stages and must work out her own strategies to move through them. In "Snake in the Mist," Joy describes the fear of the unknown, the fear of never getting better, and the fear of death. Joy is not a lightweight. She has fought and won several skirmishes with physicians. She has learned to cope in her personal and professional life, but illness has taken its toll.

Adrenaline is the fuel for the fight and serotonin the buffer of stress, but Joy has been fighting so long trying to deal with chronic pain, fatigue, doctors, and tests, her adrenaline and serotonins are low. Without these fuels, an even greater fatigue develops and Joy feels paralyzed. Some might describe Joy's state as clinical depression, but she is really experiencing the deeply rooted fears of the dark, the unknown, and of death that most of us retain from childhood. She writes, "I'm afraid of this dense dark, and I'm dismayed that I am powerless to penetrate it even slightly. I fear that there is something out there that I can't see, like a snake in the mist, coiled and waiting to strike at me. The truth is, I am just afraid."

What are your greatest fears? Is it that you can't find a doctor who will listen to you and acknowledge your suffering? Or that a curable illness is being missed? Do you fear the challenge of personal change that is required to cope and to give your body a chance to heal? Are you afraid of telling your friends that you are sick or trying to convince your family that your illness is real? Are all these fears connected to still deeper ones—the fear of death, or the fear of dependency, or the fear of suffering? Dr. Rachel Naomi Remen, author of *Kitchen Table Wisdom* [2], is frequently quoted, "Healing may not be so much about getting better, as about letting go of everything that isn't you—all of the expectations, all of the beliefs—and becoming who you are."

On the night Joy sat out on that damp, misty porch, she had just spent the evening with friends who hugged her and said the right things, but she was still alone and she needed to be. Joy needed time with herself to come to grips with her fears.

After time of reflection, Joy found that *her* deepest fear was, "I-am-afraid-I-am-going-to-die." Is this your deepest fear? Ernest Becker wrote a 1974 Pulitzer Prize winning book, *The Denial of Death*, which helps us understand that the fear of death drives many of the ways we behave as individuals and societies [3]. There is a silver lining, however. Coming through this crisis and learning to deal with your fear of death are critical to your ability to enjoy what life still has to offer, and will help prepare you for your final journey to the end of life. I predict you will look back to this phase of your illness and see the beginning of the grace you will gain as you learn to deal with these most difficult and frightening times.

DECIDE ON YOUR STRIKE ZONE AND CALL A STRIKE WHEN YOU NEED TO

In "Three Strikes," Joy is looking for a physician. She is similar to many chronically ill patients I have seen, very sensitive about being believed or being told her symptoms aren't real. It is understandably easier for doctors to deal with illnesses they can monitor with measurable laboratory tests. When presented with a patient complaining of vague symptoms that are difficult to accurately diagnose or treat, some doctors react by becoming skeptical. This skepticism says more about the doctor than the reality of the patient's symptoms. It is easy for a physician and a patient to misunderstand each other, but it is primarily the responsibility of the physician to be the listener and to acknowledge the patient's reporting and suffering. Unfortunately, there are abundant stories like Joy's about practitioners who aren't respectful listeners. If this happens to you, or if you find yourself dealing with this kind of physician, practitioner, or health care provider, let Joy's title "Three Strikes" be a reminder of three important things she does.

First, she acknowledges communication is not a perfect science and gives the doctor three chances. Second, by calling the strikes she makes it clear that she is in charge. Third, Joy decides on her own strike zone of minimally acceptable behavior, starting with calling her first strike on the doctor's chronic tardiness.

Once her batter strikes out, Joy demonstrates a willingness to move on. Looking for another physician can be risky. Patients can be perceived as doctor shopping because they didn't hear what they wanted to hear. Changing doctors can also be costly in terms of co-pays, repeat testing, time and energy, but Joy knows what is important to her and is willing to keep looking until she finds her match. She believes she has the right to choose a health care provider she can work with and trust. So do we all.

TO GET THE HELP YOU NEED, UNDERSTAND THAT YOUR MIND AND BODY ARE CONNECTED

Many patients come see me for the first time when they have had pain symptoms for many months, and are understandably discouraged, perhaps even in despair. I might start a visit like this by saying, "There are very few patients who come to see me who are not candidates for a trial of Prozac." You undoubtedly know that Prozac is an antidepressant and you may immediately feel confused and upset. Why would I say this? Do I think you are depressed? Not necessarily. Do I think your symptoms are psychological or emotional? No. So why?

Many individuals with difficult to diagnose illnesses are made to think the problem is in their heads or that they are making up symptoms to get attention. While I almost never see someone that I think is malingering, or making up symptoms, it is critical for you to understand how the mind and body do affect each other. I try to create an opportunity to discuss this without putting a person on the defensive. While my responsibility is to diagnose and treat medical conditions, I know true healing will depend on your ability to help your body to stabilize, balance, and restore. Beginning this conversation before I know you well allows me to speak in generalities, not specifically about you. You get the opportunity to understand how I think and to discuss concerns and biases you might have in a nonjudgmental way. I want to help you understand the chemical and coping aspects related to healing, and I hope this will lay the foundation for a trusting relationship with me.

I start by discussing serotonins, the natural brain chemical that is increased by Prozac and other drugs called selective serotonin reuptake inhibitors. Serotonin helps buffer all types of stress to our bodies, and it also modulates many other body and brain chemicals and immune system functions. I can summarize a vast amount of research in this area with the simple statement, "The mind and the body ARE connected." We know that frustration, anger, sleep disturbance, and reduced exercise or sunlight may reduce serotonin levels, but there are no blood tests to easily measure these effects. Sometimes only a treatment trial can tell me if your condition could be improved by boosting serotonin levels. Therefore, I may suggest you try one of these medications without diagnosing you as depressed, to see if you experience reduced symptoms or an improvement in your sense of well-being.

About thirty years after Prozac came into the market, an article was published in a leading arthritis journal that described its anti-inflammatory properties in humans and mouse models with rheumatoid arthritis. This remarkable finding further adds to the wide number of balancing affects outside the brain that serotonins and medicines like Prozac play throughout the body.

Often persons with new illnesses are more anxious about what they don't know than what they do know. Even after getting a diagnosis for their illness, individuals frequently don't know what actually caused it or what the future may hold. They describe their frustration at being unable to plan for tomorrow, or next week, or next month. They worry that they will let their families or employers down if they commit to do something, only to have their symptoms flare up so they are unable to meet that commitment. Will they be able to continue school and graduate? Are they going to lose their jobs? Will this illness become *chronic*?

Conversely, some people start to feel guilty when they have a good day and have not committed to an activity they could have performed on that day. As an illness does become chronic, feeling good can be as emotionally difficult as feeling bad. Whether to do more or to do less is a question that carries risks in both directions.

Individuals deal with the stress of illness in many different ways, but many will go through a time when they feel depressed and be overcome by a feeling of hopelessness or a loss interest in doing things. Other symptoms of depression are poor sleep, fatigue, and difficulty concentrating. In these cases, it can be hard to sort out the symptoms of illness versus the depression due to illness. Some patients create a mental barrier that allows them to deny or resist paying attention to their illness. The cost of this effort can become so overwhelming that they feel numb and fail to acknowledge they are ill at all. Psychologists describe this type of coping as *internalization* or *denial*. If hopelessness or denial leads you to a dangerous disinterest in living, then it is an important and positive next step to get professional assistance to help regain control and to find a way out of your despair. If your physician refers you to a psychologist and psychiatrist, it does not mean your illness is not real, but it may mean your illness is overwhelming and you need some help in coping with it. Studies have shown that the combination of medications to treat your symptoms and professional help in coping are more effective when combined than either one is alone.

During the *Getting Sick* phase you might also have problems in the social domains of illness—at work, with family members, and with insurance companies. It is appropriate to ask the members of your health care team to advocate for you and help educate others. Bring your family to appointments so they can understand what is going on. Some family members become overly protective, while others try too hard to solve your problems and sometimes become angry when they can't. Counselors or physicians can assist your loved ones in understanding where and how they can be most helpful. A disability counselor can help you understand your rights under the Americans with Disabilities Act of 1990 and work with your employer to prevent misunderstandings. As the saying goes, an ounce of prevention is worth a pound of cure, so it is important for you to get any help you need as soon as problems surface to ensure communication remains open and clear with family members and employers.

SEEK A DIAGNOSIS AND BEGIN TREATMENT

I have heard a number of patients interpret the term chronic illness to mean, "There's nothing to be done, so I will just have to learn to live with it on my own." This is only half true; when an illness becomes chronic, it does require learning to live with it, however it does not and should not mean living with it alone. Further, chronic doesn't mean there is no effective treatment because most of the time much can be done to ease symptoms and help the body improve balance. For example, rheumatoid arthritis is a chronic illness with many therapies, both old and new, that can bring considerable improvement to most patients and even arrest joint destruction and prevent work disability.

In order to help you during the *Getting Sick* phase, we must first try to figure out your medical diagnosis and begin a treatment plan. This can be a complex process. We just talked about symptoms caused by an understandable depression. Other symptoms can be caused by an imbalance of the immune or metabolic systems rather than by the underlying disease. So, instead of discussing all the possible diagnoses and the ways doctors think about symptoms, I want to illustrate how we can work together to improve your health and help you cope.

First, you must tell me your story. In medical school we are taught that 90% of making a diagnosis comes from the *history*, which is what we call your story. You may get tired of telling yours over and over, but it is the most important time of our work together. From your descriptions, a review of past tests and an awareness of prior physician's opinions, I look for connections and a common picture. It's like trying to put a puzzle together when there may be some pieces missing from the box. For example, not everyone develops a full-blown condition. Having a partial form of a condition may mean its symptoms are milder, but it is even more frustrating since it's harder to diagnose. Each part of your story provides a unique piece of information. As we work together, I may have to do a lot of rearranging of the puzzle pieces because the clues I find may not be specific for one disease. Many diseases and syndromes have symptoms in common, so we frequently must look closely for other clues that might lead us to a diagnosis. I am interested in your family history, the factors that aggravate or alleviate your symptoms, and even what you think might be going on. It is my job to look for patterns that could be explained by one diagnosis, and other patterns that might indicate multiple conditions that have colluded together to create an unrecognizable clinical syndrome. I even want to go back to when you were a child to see if you have had prior traumas or infections, which might have triggered a chronic process, or to see if you had an undiagnosed illness that might relate to your current problems.

Once I have your history, I will order tests. Many patients who know they are ill become frustrated when test results come back normal. We expect modern medicine to be able to identify or measure all abnormalities, but the reality is that it can't. For example, we can't yet measure whether your brain or other tissues have enough serotonin. Other factors like cytokines, the communication chemicals between immune cells, can be measured by researchers but are not routinely available for practicing physicians. Due to the fact that your illness may wax and wane, abnormalities can appear and disappear, so on any given day test results that previously showed abnormalities may return to normal.

I order more tests as I add pieces to the puzzle. These puzzle pieces include results from the first round of tests, your response to initial treatments, and your own new insights about associations between activities and symptoms. All of these factors influence the picture I see and prompt the second and third round of diagnostic tests I will order. Many common conditions present themselves in unusual ways, and conversely, some rare conditions masquerade as common. For example, celiac sprue is a condition where the immune system reacts against gluten, a protein in wheat. The classic set of symptoms for celiac disease include diarrhea. However, I have seen individuals with sprue whose major symptoms are fatigue or aching joints, or they present with asymptomatic osteoporosis. These patients won't complain first of diarrhea. In order to solve the mystery of their illness, I have to consider the less common complications of celiac illness before I would think to order celiac tests. This process takes time and care on the part of the patient and the physician, constantly relooking at the whole picture to see if a new pattern is revealing itself.

Sometimes patients respond to one of my therapy suggestions by saying, "I've tried that before and it didn't work." They have lost faith not only in a treatment, but also in the doctor who first ordered it. Sometimes patients provide a long list of remedies they have tried, and are unwilling to try again. These repeated failures have left them feeling stalled, frustrated, and hopeless. However, just because a therapy did not work once, doesn't mean that it should go on a black list of treatments never to be tried again. When it joins other therapies as part of a new effort, at a different time, and with a new team, the results may be more successful. It is like making vegetable soup. There are as many different ways to make the soup as there are cooks and ingredients.

BUILD A SUPPORTIVE HEALTH CARE TEAM AND BECOME A TEAM PLAYER

A trusted physician doesn't have to meet all your needs, but he or she can be the leader to help you build your team and advocate for you. Other doctors or therapists will give you medicines, provide hands-on care, offer injections, or suggest surgery, but they all need to understand and integrate into one overall treatment plan led by your *principal* physician.

There are two things you have the right to expect and demand from every practitioner who treats you:

1. Open and detailed discussions with you, answering all your questions and helping you feel heard and in control.
2. Consistent communication with your principal physician and active integration of his or her recommendations into your comprehensive care plan.

This is what integrated care means—many clinicians and professionals working together to help you develop one roadmap for care. This roadmap should be updated continuously as you move through the phases and cover all four domains of life that your illness impacts. The four domains are:

- physical or medical
- emotional or psychological
- family or social
- spiritual or existential

As your principal physician, or team leader, this four-part perspective helps me think about the types of treatments and support I need to offer, what your other providers are offering, and in what areas you might need to improve your skill and confidence.

Another way I look at integrating care among your many providers is to divide your therapies into three parts: Those done TO YOU; the self-care and therapies that involve YOU FOR YOU; and the strategies that involve YOU AND OTHERS. For each pill, procedure, or hands-on therapy prescribed by your practitioners, the TO YOU, I suggest that you identify and write down a parallel YOU FOR YOU self-care activity that you will engage in to complement it. And then, for each phase of your care, consider how you can modify your relationship with others so they can better help you. These are the YOU AND OTHERS conversations with loved ones, friends, or work associates that can be stressful, but are necessary.

Remember the *Stuck Car* story and my comment that you may need to learn to drive differently? This means that you must consider and discuss with others how your conventional wisdom may not be working anymore. Do you need to learn how to experience and understand your body differently? What behaviors do you need to change and how can this help you? This responsibility on your part speaks to the reality that your doctor can't do everything, and that you need to be an active member of the team, too. During the next phase of *Being Sick*, you will learn that you are not only on the team, but need to be at the center, like the hub of a wheel with many spokes of support.

Phase II
Being Sick

Pain

As a child, I dreamed of a life on the stage. I took ballet lessons for decades and even became a member of a civic ballet company as a teen. I also took voice lessons and sang in the chorus from elementary through high school. When I went to college I majored in Fine Arts until the realities of earning a living trumped my dream of a stage career. I switched to Education and as a teacher tried my best to transfer what I knew about engaging an audience to a room full of restless kids.

I was in my late 30s when I moved to San Juan Island, Washington, and the dreams of my youth finally came true. Our small island had a thriving community theater and anyone could audition to act and sing, even direct and choreograph. For the first few years that we lived there, I eagerly signed up for everything, until I became too ill to participate.

Now, I miss the camaraderie of the cast and crew, the smell of the stage boards, and the feel of the heavy, black velvet wing curtain. I used to pull that curtain to my face and peer through a little tear in the fabric to check the size of the house before the five-minutes-until-curtain call. My special blue plastic makeup box now sits on a shelf gathering dust, the eye shadow and lip color pots dry and cracked inside.

One day, a director at our theater sought me out. He hadn't seen me around for a while and must not have remembered I am sick. He asked if I would consider being in *Chapter Two*, an upcoming play, and offered me the part of Jenny Malone, the female lead. Before moving to the island, this director had a long, distinguished career in the movies and is a man of his era with a John Wayne voice and Jimmy Stewart charm. Since retiring from the movie business, he's been willing to lend his gifts to our amateur productions and it would be an honor to work with him. In a flash, the activity monitor that has kept me operating safely within my little sick box blew a fuse.

I'm pretty stable, I told myself. Most days I can keep my symptoms under control. Maybe I have it in me to do this now. After all, the aging director can get himself into the theater to do his job; surely I could muster up enough energy to get in there and do mine. Bedsides, Jenny Malone is a great part. She's an energetic, positive woman; that would be good for me. We negotiated.

"Can rehearsals be limited to two hours?" I asked.

"Sure," he answered.

"And not every single day."

"No, certainly not."

"If I get sick, would it be okay if I missed rehearsal, maybe just a time or two?"

"Of course," he assured me. "Don't worry, dear, we'll get along just fine."

For the first few weeks of rehearsals we did get along just fine, in our slow, halting way. But my activity monitor, the one with the blown fuse? Well, it blew right before I thought about the part that comes *after* rehearsal—The Performances.

The week before opening night is called Tech Week. Rehearsals are long and grueling, often lasting well past midnight. The scenes, costume, and set changes are timed and then must be done again in less time, and again in still less time. Technical cues for sound and lighting are checked and rechecked. Props are placed exactly on their marks, represented by colored tape on the stage. Actors must stand silently on their colored marks for what seems like hours, while the lighting is adjusted to complement our new costumes and make up.

I began the week in bad shape, bone tired, beyond tired. I felt like I was moving through cotton, muffled. The ache that started in my hips and spine had spread into all of my joints and deep into my muscles and through my nerves and onto my skin. When George reached out to touch my arm, I felt bruised. I was, in fact, one big bruise.

I had so many costume changes a dressing room was built for me in the wings and I had a helper who waited while I changed my clothes, then handed me my next hat, purse, and collection of jewelry. While changing my costume, I had to loudly deliver lines to actors waiting for me to return to the stage quickly, and on cue. At the end of the play, I had to hit George, hard, and cry on cue as our marriage fell apart and my heart broke. There were hundreds of lines to remember, and I'd learned them all, but pain was filling up my mind like water flooding the cabin of a sinking ship. I was drowning in pain and there was little room left for words. It became clear to me that I would not make it through the three-week run of this play unless I found a way to control the consuming pain.

The night before final dress rehearsal, we ran the whole play without interruption for the first time. Shortly before curtain, in desperation, I took a prescription Vicodin, a narcotic pain tablet. I'd had a bottle of Vicodin in my medicine cabinet for months, and I knew the instructions on its proper use, but I'd avoided taking it. I was scared of narcotics, scared of addiction, and scared of losing control. Before this day, I'd opted to take an over-the-counter pain medication and endure the pain because I would rather pull the covers over my head and suffer than submit to the risks I associated with narcotics. This time I couldn't hide under the covers.

It was a miracle. I took one Vicodin and sailed effortlessly through the run. Well, maybe I did miss my exact mark on the stage occasionally, and I recall almost falling off my little ottoman during an impassioned speech. In fact, I think I might even have dropped a line or two, once or twice, but I'd been saved. I had no pain, so I had no problem. My performance was delivered through a lovely, soft, muted haze.

After rehearsal, the cast assembled on the stage to receive the customary director's notes. He sat in the shadows, three rows from the rear of the auditorium.

"Joy, dear, Jenny seemed a little off tonight, a little flat. Not quite up to snuff."

"I, uh, I had to take some pain medication tonight," I stammered.

"Really? Well, dear, will you be taking it again?"

Damn, damn, damn. "I, I'm not sure. I'm working it out. Don't worry."

"Well then, that's fine, dear."

The stage manager did not accept my explanation so readily. Her name was Melissa, but we called her, for good reason, Militia. She confronted me the second I stepped offstage. "What in heaven's name did you take? Give it to me, all of it. What if you lose your footing, fall off the apron, and into the pit? I'm responsible for you!"

I was ashamed and obediently prepared a sample of my pain killing stash for Militia. I used an aqua pill container that had four cubicles, each one with a little pop-top lid. I filled the first cubicle with Extra Strength Tylenol tablets, the second with Tylenol 3, which contains Codeine. I filled the other two with as many Vicodin as I could cram in. We agreed Militia would keep these locked in her stage manager's toolbox, to dole out to me upon request.

Although I understood Militia's concern and her responsibility to monitor the cast, this agreement scared me and I felt trapped. If I didn't take any pain medication at all, I feared she would still have to catch me as I fell into the pit. If I took a lightweight tablet like Extra Strength Tylenol, it would mute my current level of pain about as effectively as a fog bank quiets a foghorn. I slept on the problem and the next day I decided to try a different approach. I took another Vicodin, but earlier, at four in the afternoon, hours before I needed to perform. Then I got into bed and rested quietly until 6:30 when I left home for the theater. I was sober enough to remember to tell Militia what I had done. By curtain at eight, I'd ascended through la-la-land and was on the plateau of the drug. I didn't feel sedated, but was still pain free. I had both a brain and a memory. I could keep my balance and remember my lines. The director had his Jenny back.

After rehearsal, Militia posted a large sign on my dressing-room mirror: *Always take pain medication* four hours *before curtain.*

And so I did, before every performance for the next three weekends.

Chapter Two was a big hit. To be honest, in my small, supportive community, every show is a hit, but still, the cast was thrilled. On closing night we got a standing ovation and I was handed an armload of flowers from my dear husband, who was eagerly anticipating the resumption of the home-cooked meals he'd been missing. I would be happy to oblige him, once I slept for about a month.

The next week, the Vicodin went back on the shelf, no longer needed, at least not so often, but rebalancing my symptoms and refilling my energy tank took as long as the run of the play. My short avocation as a chronically ill actor ended with this role as I've not come across another part I feel I'm capable of doing, or worth the risk to everyone else.

I paid a high price to be Jenny Malone in *Chapter Two* and if I hadn't discovered a way to manage the pain she caused me, the whole production might have paid a high price, too. Still, I'm forever grateful to Jenny because she taught me a lot. For one thing, I now know to always have on hand many kinds of pain medication. I keep it everywhere—in my purse, in my overnight bag, in my desk drawer—just in case. I've worked with my doctors and on my own to make sure I know how to use each kind of medication, when to use it, how it will affect me, and for how long. Although at times I still have very bad pain, it has never again consumed me for weeks on end as it did during the rehearsals for *Chapter Two*. Nor do I suffer for days in bed, cut off from my life by pain. Now I know how to treat the pain. Thanks to Jenny Malone, I can sense the pain coming, like the low whistle of a train in the distance, and I've learned how to do something about it before it runs me over.

Bravo to that.

Disabled, But Not Invalid

The phone rings down the hall. I dread answering it. I also dread getting the mail each day. After months of agonizing soul-searching and the gradual, painful acceptance that I am not going to get well and can no longer effectively serve my clients, I've stopped working and made a claim for long-term disability. I first signed up for this insurance when I was a young teacher and an insurance representative said to me, "You should consider getting long-term disability as well as life insurance. The chances of becoming disabled are far greater and more devastating than premature death."

Since then my employers have always offered it and I've always purchased it, never realizing that someday I'd actually have to make the claim, or the torment I'd feel in reaching that decision. Nor did I ever suspect how badly I would be treated by the insurer when I did exercise my contract. Now, when the phone rings, or the mail is delivered, it is often a message from my disability insurer containing a veiled attack or threat, or an outright accusation that I am a fraud.

A fraud! How dare they? I am determined to prove my integrity to them, until my husband delivers a little truth serum. I am being too sensitive, too accommodating, and far too cooperative, he says. The insurer doesn't care about my ethics, or about the reality of my illness. "The business plan of a disability insurer is simple," he says. "They collect premiums and deny claims. That's the way they make a profit." In order to effectively deny claims, the company must develop a culture that supports the notion that all claims are fraudulent and they can prove it. My husband has warned me that any information I give the insurer that is not required by contract will be used against me if at all possible. Over these last months, I have come to believe he is right. I am wary and frightened of these people and their business plan and what it portends for me.

I answer the phone. "Hello."

"Joy Selak, please."

"Speaking." I know from her voice that this is my own personal Senior Risk Specialist. I also know I am the risk that she specializes in.

"Good morning, Joy. This is your own personal Senior Risk Specialist. How are we feeling today?"

"We are feeling all right." This is always a hard question for me to answer. My instinct is to say, "Fine, thank you," no matter how I feel. Or worse, "I'm having a really great day and I'm glad just to be alive!" But I know these responses are inappropriate in this context. Besides, I suspect the call is being recorded.

"So," she chirps, "have you been on any nice trips lately? I seem to remember you have a boat. I remember having a boat when I was young. I have some wonderful memories of the boat trips we took in the summer."

I lie down on the bed next to the phone. I don't know what this is about, but I can tell it's going to take a while. "We go out on our boat occasionally."

"Boy, I remember loading and unloading the boat, what a lot of work that was! That must be a lot of work for you, too, I'll bet."

"Mostly my husband does it."

"Wow. That must be a lot of work for him. Does he do it all, every single bit?"

"Sometimes I do a little."

"Gee, it must be hard for you to lift and carry all those supplies. I remember how hard it was for me, carrying all those supplies up and down the dock, back and forth."

"We have a cart."

"So, you can pull the cart. That must help. We didn't have a cart for our boat."

I can't stand it anymore. "You know, I'm a little tired. I need to rest now. Is there something specific you wanted?"

"Of course, I'm so sorry. You go rest now, but before you hang up I should tell you we've been doing just a little bit of surveillance on you, which is completely within our legal rights in order to effectively manage our risk. We feel you may be capable of substantially more activity than you have reported. We will be sending our surveillance tapes to your doctor for his review, and then we'll be talking about how you can return to work really soon. I hope you have a great day, now. I just wanted to let you know."

I start to shake before I even hang up the phone. What did they catch me doing on their surveillance tape? I remember one night I sat out on the porch and smoked a cigarette. I've never told Dr. Overman that I am an occasional secret cigarette smoker. Did they film that? Have I done anything else really bad? I frantically search my mind for every good day I've had lately. Did I ever leap into the air, skip down a sidewalk, dance cheek to cheek? Did I offload the boat?

Panicked, I call my husband. He says thoughtfully, "Why don't we get a copy of their surveillance documents and see for ourselves what they have? We have the right to do so." Good idea.

It takes a long time to receive the videos and transcripts. It seems our request is very uncommon, and therefore must be carefully cleared by the insurer's entire legal department, twice. The delay is also complicated by Dr. Overman's uncommon refusal to view the tapes at all on this first request. He asserts that he is quite competent to diagnose thousands of patients every year without doing surveillance on any of them. He says the tapes are legal data, not medical data. Later he did review them and found nothing unexpected, but by then I had confessed to the occasional cigarette.

As my husband and I wait for the tapes, we use the time to review our history with the disability insurer. After I filed my initial claim, it took seven months before I began to receive payments. Even then the company "reserved the right" to arbitrarily cancel my income based on results of their ongoing investigation of me, which had no deadline at all. Later, they abruptly reduced my monthly payments based on their unsubstantiated claim that my employer had overstated my earnings. Before they admitted to their error, they were in arrears to me by more than a thousand dollars. What if I had been a single parent with young children to care for during this time? How would my family have survived?

We remember the Federal Express envelope that was left at our front door. The letter inside announced I must attend a Mandatory Independent Medical Exam in Seattle, scheduled without my knowledge or consent for five days after its arrival. The letter threatened, in bold print, to terminate my benefits if I didn't attend the appointment as scheduled. I don't know what the consequences would have been if we'd been out on the boat that week. Then the insurer objected to paying my travel expenses to the exam because they asserted it wasn't their fault that I chose to live in a rural area without a practicing neuro-psychologist. We argued that it wasn't my fault I had become disabled either, and I didn't choose my home in anticipation of that tragedy. In time, we learned that paying my travel expenses was, in fact, the insurer's obligation.

The exam lasted eight grueling hours and involved dozens of tests. After I left the neuropsychologist's office, I was required to complete several additional questionnaires at my hotel that night and return them the next morning. After delivering the documents, I returned home, exhausted, to await the report. When the thirty-page document arrived, the doctor stated that in his opinion I had a *somatoform disorder*, meaning I was overly concerned with being ill and needed psychoanalysis. I was flabbergasted. I thought I was sent to this man specifically to dis-cuss my illness; how could he conclude I was overly concerned with it?

My husband reminded me that according to my disability insurance policy, a mental health diagnosis pays twenty percent less against earned income than a physical disability. My insurer was once again employing their risk management strategy, hop-ing to increase their revenues by reducing mine. Dr. Overman expertly countered the report, analyzing the test results for data that were discounted or ignored, and citing numerous research studies to support my physical disability.

We remember the independent consultant the insurance company hired and sent to our home to interview me and assess my function in my home setting. When we confessed to him the difficulties we'd experienced with the insurer, he confessed to us that statistically, out of all the people who purchase disability insurance, only 5% ever make a claim. Of that 5%, only 5% are found to be fraudulent. He tells us that insurers base their examination of every claim as if it were one of those 1/4 of 1% possibly fraudulent claims. With a little quick math, we calculate his statistics would indicate that in my company of 10,000 employees, assuming 6,000 purchase disability insurance, only 300 of those employees will ever make a claim. Of those 300, 15 might prove to be fraudulent. So, I am being treated this way because this insurer is convinced I might be one of *15* bad guys out of *6,000* good guys. This also means that about 5,700 of my colleagues are paying this company monthly premiums in good faith and will get absolutely nothing in return, except some peace of mind.

I call my corporate Human Resources Department to check on these assumptions. I am told that in the entire firm there are actually only two active disability claims with the insurer. The other was filed by a double amputee diabetic, bound to a wheelchair, and his claim was also being vigorously challenged. It seems he was once recorded on the phone saying, "I have to know if you are going to approve this claim. I have children and can't wait any longer; I'm going to have to find a way to support them." This desperate statement was used as proof this man was capable of returning to work.

By the time the surveillance tapes finally arrive, we have become very angry and very weary of this whole process. Worse, we wonder how I can ever get well when I have to spend so much time proving I am sick.

The videos are shocking only in their uselessness. They show me walking up a dock with my dog, my mother, and an 83-year-old friend. They document the existence of my house, mailbox, car, truck, and boat. They show the studio where I go to receive massage therapy and the pool where I take a water therapy class. I can tell where the detective must have stationed himself on the hill above our bare-windowed country home, armed with a camera and telephoto lens, and filmed me as I walked from the back door to the car. Did he also film me in the bathroom or bedroom, just for fun? Being spied on this way is a violation, but nevertheless I'm glad to have the tapes, because both the dog and the 83-year-old friend have died and this film will be a treasured record of them.

The written transcripts are more shocking because the hostility and bias of the surveillance officer is unleashed without accompanying videos to substantiate his claims. For example, he attests that items he sees me carry off the boat, which he calls a yacht, *appear* to be very heavy and yet I lift them with ease. He disputes the symptoms I have reported by stating my walk is brisk and fluid and I do not *appear* to be in any pain. He writes that after observing me enter and leave several stores while holding a cup of coffee I don't *appear* to ever stop to go to the bathroom. He documents that he followed me all over the island where I live, as well as to Seattle and back and actually complains that he could not get access to me in the hotel where I stayed. This out of town surveillance occurred, coincidentally, on the day of my appointment with the neuropsychologist. How can a doctor be labeled an Independent Medical Examiner when he coordinates his medical appointment with an insurer's secret surveillance of the patient?

The surveillance report goes on to say I consistently drive five miles over the speed limit, use every opportunity to shop, and do not control my dog. While spying through the window of a restaurant where my husband and I are having dinner with friends, he observes that I do most of the talking and look animated and wave my arms as if I am having a lot of fun. These insights occur over five separate days during which he calls my house and my hotel room nine different times, under pretense, as early as 6:30 in the morning, to determine if I am there.

My husband looks up from his reading and says, "I don't think it's legal to call people under false pretenses."

The mood shifts.

We contact our sheriff and he confirms it is indeed illegal to use the telephone under false pretenses; it is considered harassment.

All our pent-up feelings of helplessness and rage erupt. We file a complaint with the sheriff, who is outraged and immediately joins our team. He sends an officer to our only local private investigator's home to warn him that criminal charges will be filed if he breaks any law while doing surveillance of me. The police put a trace on our telephone. We file complaints with the Federal Communications Commission and the state insurance commissioner. We write formal complaint letters, with our long lists of grievances, to the CEO of the insurance company, to every representative of the company who has been rude to us, to their department heads and to my own personal Senior Risk Specialist. The floor is littered with drafts and labels and extra copies. Soon we are laughing and congratulating each other as each envelope is sealed.

Then my husband comes up with the pièce de résistance. He suggests we have our attorney prepare an affidavit giving him complete power of attorney over all my insurance matters. I sign it and then he instructs the insurer never to contact me by phone or by mail again. They must deal only with him, a fully functioning, alert, competent and healthy person. That night we sleep deeply, as if we have at last received a commuted sentence for a crime we never committed.

Despite our tirade, the surveillance doesn't stop for a while, and neither do the demands that I attend independent medical exams with hired guns whose leading credential is they don't believe the illnesses I have even exist. But now we have become much better at managing this system. We set our own conditions for participation in the exams. If I am not available, it must be rescheduled. My husband always comes with me as an observer. We stop the process when I tire or feel too ill to continue. My husband calls the insurance company every six months and demands to see any new surveillance material. We question their every move that is in any way unresponsive or disrespectful to me. We remind ourselves of all the premiums we have paid, and he continues to pay, in good faith, so that we could collect payments in the event such a terrible tragedy as this should befall us. Now, secure in the knowledge that these people owe us, we shamelessly demand what we are owed.

At our house there may live a person who is disabled, but no one here is invalid.

The Ladies Who Lunch

E ach table at the ladies' spring luncheon and fashion show is draped to the floor with a leaf-green tablecloth and topped with a white wicker basket overflowing with tulips, daffodils, crocus, and iris. The porcelain plates have silver rims and there are pink napkins folded like origami and tucked into long-stemmed wine glasses. A complicated array of flatware frames the plates and on each one sits an embossed calling card with guest names hand-written in calligraphy. I wander the room from table to vibrant table, searching for the card that bears my name.

At this time of day, midday, I enjoy my few hours of peak energy and try to use the brief window of time to take a walk, keep appointments, or run necessary errands. I don't usually spend this precious time, as I will today, at a fashion show eating lunch with nine women I barely know. When at last I discover my place, I feel tired just looking at the ten chairs ringing the table, anticipating the amount of talking that will go on for the next few hours. I have learned that talking is very high on my list of energy-draining activities, which is not to say I have quit talking, but I have definitely curtailed talking. I decide to go to the bathroom before I sit down and use the time to try and calm the anxiety that I feel. Too many times in social situations like

47

this, people who don't even know me have made hurtful, even cruel, comments when they find out about my illness. I've had total strangers blame me for getting sick and then further blame me for being unable to get well, and it seems the people who know the least about the subject can be the most judgmental. My patience has grown very, very thin on this matter. On the other hand, this luncheon is a fundraiser for a worthy cause, a good friend asked me to attend, and I haven't been out in a while, so I'll hope for the best. I return to the table, the last to arrive. I take my seat, and we begin the ritual of sharing vital statistics—our names, where we are from, our line of work, if we work, and what our husbands do, if there are husbands.

First I greet Joan, the only person I know well at all. She is a descendent of one of the families who settled the island generations ago and opened the hardware store. They still own and operate it to this day. I don't know why merely staying in the same place for generations makes a family so important, but it does on this island. Then Alice introduces her friend Beverly who is visiting from California. Both women are in their seventies. They were college roommates and have traveled to see each other every year for more than forty years.

To my immediate left is Angela, a newcomer to the island, and an attractive, thirty-something high-tech professional. She cashed in her company stock options and retired to our island with her husband and two young children to kayak and hike and live the good life. She is fresh, athletic, and bright and doesn't know a soul here yet. To my right is Madge who is suffering from early dementia. Madge is often seen shoplifting trinkets from the drugstore and stuffing them into her oversized coat pockets, but she is never apprehended for her crimes because the druggist simply calls her husband once a week with the list of items to be returned. Madge has been a beloved, valuable citizen of our small community and I appreciate that she is offered this dignity.

Ginny is over for the week from a nearby island and I have heard through the grapevine that she is dating a wealthy local widower. She tells us he is off playing golf today. Finally, there are three visitors from the mainland, Betty, Sue, and Barb. They are here for a week in a vacation condo and needed something to do while their husbands are off fishing. That makes all ten of us and I am already having brain fog trying to keep track of them all. I look around the table and attempt to memorize names— Joan, Alice and Beverly, Angela left, Madge right, Ginny and Betty-Sue-Barb. That's only nine. Oh, me. Of course.

The conclusion of our introductions coincides with the first course of lunch service, and then the fashion show begins. Between courses and models I strike up a conversation with Angela, the young retired technical professional on my left, while trying hard to include Madge, the older shoplifting amateur to my right. I know the lapses in the program that allow for these brief conversations occur because the models we are seeing on the runway are not models at all, but local women enlisted for the event. I can visualize them hopping about on one leg in the bathroom, squeezing into girdles, running their panty hose and consumed with the stress of momentary stardom. I know because I've been there and done that, equally awkwardly.

I tell Angela I was once a stockbroker on the island and the company stock that allowed her to retire and move to paradise was also very good to my former clients. After expressing her surprise that a big national firm like mine has an office on the island, she asks why I am no longer a stockbroker. Now, I could have simply said, "I retired, too," but no-o-o-o, I had to say, "Well, I came down with this chronic illness, so I had to quit working."

"Really? You don't *look* sick."

I was just starting to like Angela, but I really, really hate it when people say you don't *look* sick. It's like they think I'm faking, or that looking well is some compensation for being sick. Actually, I wish I did look sick, just for the sake of credibility, like a little kid who marks a wound with a brightly colored bandage.

Then Madge, who has been ignored for too long, punches my arm and says, "Sick, who's sick? I am *not* sick."

"Is someone sick?" Joan perks up. "Here, I can tell you where the bathroom is, although it's a bit overcrowded with models right now. There is another bathroom you can use, right around the outside of this building."

"Joy says she is sick, but not that kind of sick," explains Angela with a warm smile, "and she was just about to tell me about it."

Great. I pan the nine faces waiting expectantly for my answer. Well, eight, I can't count Madge, who is busy putting her salad fork in her coat pocket. I make a mental note to tell the club manager so he can call her husband.

"I, uh, I have a chronic illness. It's called mixed, or undifferentiated, connective tissue disease." I decide, as usual, to leave out the bladder disease considering we are all eating.

"Those words are too big for me. What do you have in English?" asks Beverly from the Bay Area.

"In English, I have pain, and fatigue, and an over-active immune system."

Alice points at me with her fork, "You know I have a cousin in Poughkeepsie who has celiac disease and she went to a doctor who put her on this really strict diet where she can't eat any bread, or cake, or basically anything good. But now she's a whole lot better. Have you tried that diet?"

"No, I haven't, but you see, Alice, I don't have celiac disease."

"I know, but have you tried it? It might help!"

This is what people do. Right out of the gate, they try to fix you, even if they don't know what they are talking about. If you won't immediately accept their fix, they are even more certain they have the answer.

"Like I said before, I don't have celiac disease."

Then from the Betty-Sue-Barb side of the table I overhear the comment, "Well, I think all illnesses are psychosomatic, don't you?"

Is she asking this of me, the sick person? I pretend I don't hear, but if things run true to form, next they will start talking about God.

"I think illness is God's way of teaching us a lesson," adds Sue.

"And in His love, He never gives us more than we can handle," is Barb's sweetly spoken final embellishment.

Please, if there is a God, can he shut these people up? I glance at my water glass and am actually tempted to whack it across the table and into their laps. Instead, I look around the table and say pointedly, "I take your comments to mean that none of you has ever *had* a chronic illness?"

"Well, to me you don't look sick," repeats Angela and I see from her kind expression that she thinks this is a compliment.

I take a deep breath and try to locate my polite, socially acceptable self, "Well, yes, thank you. I get lots of rest."

Then Ginny the merry widow, having overheard my comment that I can no longer work, whines, "You are so lucky you don't *have* to work. My husband left me with very little money, and I *have* to work unless, of course, I marry again. I wish I could be a little bit sick so I didn't *have* to work."

"I like to work and I would work if I could," I protest. "And besides, I'm not a *little* bit sick." Ginny responds with a disbelieving shrug. This really sets me off and I add, too loudly. "I *miss* working!"

My tone so startles Ginny that she drops her fork and a big smear of chicken salad falls onto the front of her blouse. She turns to Joan and asks in a quivering voice, "Where did you say that ladies' room was located?"

After she leaves, the waiters begin to clear the salad plates and deliver the main course. We stop talking and I have a brief moment of hope that this conversation might be over, but as soon as we are all served, Joan picks up the ball. "From what I've heard around town, Joy, this has been going on for quite a while. Why don't you get a good doctor and get yourself well?"

"I have changed doctors—more than once—I have good doctors—what have you heard around town?"

"Not for me to say, but anyway, if it was my life, I'd get myself a new doctor and get over it."

"I don't need a new doctor—I have an excellent doctor." I stop, take a breath and try to calm down. I feel like I'm bobbing around like one of those dashboard dolls with its head on a spring. "Look, Joan, my illness is chronic. Chronic. That means there is *no known cure.*"

"Well, still, I think if you really wanted to you could get well. Sometimes people stay sick because there's some payoff to it, you know. How's your marriage, by the way?"

Oh, for heaven's sake. "My marriage is great, Joan. And the *doctor* who told me my illness was chronic was actually *qualified* to make that diagnosis, but thanks anyway."

"Whatever." Joan turns away from me dismissively. "Oh, welcome back, Ginny dear. Did you find that ladies' room all right?"

51

Ginny takes her seat quietly, a large water stain bleeding dark blue across the front of her light blue silk blouse, which I find shamelessly gratifying.

Alice carries on, "Have you been under a lot of stress, dear? I hear that stress can cause a lot of these illnesses."

I lean forward and declare to all of them, too loudly. "I am *completely* relaxed! I am not under *any* stress!"

I sit back and nine faces stare at me in shock. They actually look frightened, as if one more outburst from me will cause them to collectively dive under the table for protection. As I take in their silent, frozen faces, I am jerked back to my senses. What am I doing? These women can't possibly know what it's like to be me—sentenced to live in a prison of illness, without hope of healing, surrounded by judgmental skeptics. They don't know a thing about me, or my life—not anything at all. A ten way conversation at a charity luncheon and fashion show is not the appropriate time to teach them.

"I'm, I'm sorry," I say. "I'm just tired. I think I need to go home and rest now." I push back my chair, stand and say politely, "It was nice to meet all of you ladies. I hope you enjoy the rest of your day."

I turn and start my lonely walk across the room. I can hear the murmur of low voices behind me as the conversation goes on without me, most likely about me. What do I need to learn here? These women aren't really malicious, they are just ignorant. In fact, I am the one who has behaved badly because I know better. And my defensiveness hasn't done anything to increase their understanding, or reduce their mistrust of people like me. The only thing I've accomplished is to completely wear myself out.

As I step outside and into the fresh air I vow that next time, next time, I'll do better. I will try to understand that people act this way because they are afraid of illness. If they can convince themselves I brought this all on myself, then they can believe it will never happen to them. If I'm honest, I probably did the same thing myself, before I knew better. I was changed by illness, not fairness. Next time, I won't take their comments as a personal assault. Next time, I will be patient and try to help them understand.

If I try harder, maybe next time they will, too.

Dr. Overman on Being Sick: The Athlete and the Coach

In the first phase, *Getting Sick*, I wrote that as a patient, you must build a health care team and become a team player. Ultimately you must become the hub of your team. Let's take that analogy to the next level now that you have entered a new phase: *Being Sick*. While you still may not fully understand your diagnosis, or have an adequate explanation from medical science as to why you became ill, once you enter the *Being Sick* phase, you are well into caring for yourself. If I were your doctor, we might still have many therapy combinations to try, and I would not have given up hope that you might attain a remission. I'd ask how you would like to work with me during this phase of your illness.

You are learning your illness is not going away, at least not for now, so managing it is not a sprint, but a long-distance journey. This race must be run with the determination of a highly trained athlete so you can effectively cope with the limitations of illness, the physical ups and downs and the roadblocks of the health care system. On our team, I like to think of your role as the athlete and your providers as your coaches. While Joy, like many of my patients, uses the term *partnership* as the ideal goal of the doctor/patient relationship, I feel this does not fully acknowledge my professional duties. In acute care, patients expect the doctor to quickly provide the therapeutic answer through surgery or medications. Treating chronic illness requires an ongoing commitment from both you and me. My goal is to work with you over time so that, like a world-class athlete, you can learn to perform at your peak capacity. And like a coach who is in this relationship for the long haul, I have no quick fixes. My job is more than giving answers. I need to educate, counsel, and encourage you to set goals and implement a personal care program, as well as take appropriate medications.

What coaching do you need in the treatment of pain, a symptom common to so many invisible illnesses? In order to help you, I would need to see how you perform and know what your goals are. Since this may change from month to month, I would ask you at each visit to fill out the same questionnaire. I use this method to gather information about your current symptoms and function and to track progress toward your goals over time. While a few of you might groan at all the extra writing each visit, I would ask you to consider the difference between watching a painter at work, and seeing the finished painting. It takes a long time for a painter to finish a work of art, or for you tell me everything that is on your mind. Just as a completed painting can evoke a very quick response, the picture provided on the detailed questionnaire helps me know at a glance where you are on the illness journey and how you are doing in many domains. Also, by looking first at your complete *illness* picture, I can understand where you are in the broader dimension of *wellness*. Once I have this general picture, your specific story will highlight and prioritize the issues important to my thinking. I can now more quickly zero in on specific questions you have rather than spending too much of our visit helping you to paint the picture. So while maybe you didn't like the questionnaire at the beginning of the visit, I promise you it will help prevent the frustration you might have had at the end of the visit—feeling I hadn't acknowledged all that you were experiencing or failed to answer all your questions.

During this phase of *Being Sick*, my goal is to help you gain *confidence* in managing your illness: adjusting medications, improving exercise, managing diet and stress, and increasing work and social activities where possible. I recognize the illness journey is also challenging for those who care about you. They also face lost dreams and feelings of anger, fear, guilt, or helplessness. Their valued functions or roles may have to change, so it is my job to make sure you have support in dealing with these important areas. Teamwork, taking action, regaining control, and finding a balance are some of the necessary ingredients for navigating *Being Sick*. Let's review what Joy did and I'll again offer some tips that might help you on your way.

LEARN TO MANAGE YOUR PAIN

Through her illness experience, Joy had already learned to listen more closely to her body, to pace herself and not fight all her battles alone. So, even though she knows she will risk flare-ups of pain and fatigue, she decides to take a part in a play, reasoning she can handle it and the cost will be balanced by the nutrition to her spirit. She learns that in order to participate, she must overcome her bias against pain medications and learn to use these drugs effectively and responsibly. As a result of this experience, Joy realizes greater function, freedom, and self-confidence.

Let's talk about pain, which left uncontrolled can become self-perpetuating. I like to say that chronic pain can stretch the nervous system so that previously benign stimuli can become painful. This stretch phenomenon is called *neuroplasticity*, and pain triggered by nonpainful stimuli is called *allodynia*. An experiment was conducted that may help you understand the concept. A subject was pricked with a needle in the forearm, and flinched. But when an area two inches away from the needle stick was touched with cotton, the subject did not flinch, because it was not painful. After multiple needle sticks, the second spot, two inches away, did become painful at the mere touch of cotton. This phenomenon helps explain some of the widespread pain and tenderness that often develops in chronic pain syndromes like fibromyalgia, which may develop after inflammatory arthritis or tendinitis begin the pain. Joy describes such flares as feeling like she is one big bruise. She says it hurts when another actor touches her arm. Joy has allodynia.

Now that you have a little basic education about pain, I would ask you to tell me how and when your pain first began. By examining the initial event, even if it were long ago, we might find clues to imbalances where specific repairs are needed, through surgery or physical therapy. Next we would look at your daily habits. For example, too much coffee or cola can result in poor sleep, anxiety, and increased blood pressure. Poor posture or movement patterns can cause re-injury. Anger or fear can increase adrenaline and alter temperature, pulse, blood pressure, and immune system function. We may want to address workplace or family problems. Your frustration with your pain can make it difficult to recognize that any of these factors could be fueling the pain syndrome. Practices such as meditation and cognitive counseling may help you understand your emotional responses, change them as needed, and better manage your pain. Other strategies can help you reduce pain without medications. Remember when you were a child and asked your mom or dad to rub your "owies?" You instinctively knew that rubbing the painful area would make it all better. This is because touch can block the pain stimuli that travel through the spinal cord. A variety of modalities may work in a similar fashion, such as acupuncture, a transcutaneous nerve stimulator, ice and heat therapy, and massage. Movement therapies such as yoga help for a variety of reasons, directly and indirectly altering pain triggers, tissue healing, and pain perception. Conversely, hiding under the covers for days on end, as Joy did for so long, will do little to help.

Next, I'd want to talk to you about a number of medications that can also help block the pain stimuli. These medications, called *neuromodulators*, work on different parts of the nervous system, but remain categorized by their first FDA-approved use: antidepressant, anti-seizure, sleep, muscle relaxant, and narcotic medications. The use of narcotics for pain management has become a complex issue because of misinformation and some abuse regarding them. But, as Joy learned, narcotic medication can very effectively control acute and recurrent pain, allowing you to focus on rehabilitation efforts, reduce the energy required to battle the pain, gain more confidence about making social commitments, and possibly prevent a longer term pain syndrome.

Your body's natural narcotics are called *endorphins* and, in response to a number of stimuli, they are normally produced by the pituitary gland and the hypothalamus. You have probably heard runners describe how they were able to work through fatigue and pain and continue to run beyond their usual limit. This has been described as an *endorphin high* or a *runner's high* since they frequently describe feeling almost euphoric. Other brain chemicals such as serotonin, dopamine, and epinephrine may also work with the endorphins to allow people to continue pushing the body long after they thought they could go no further. You can imagine how this defense mechanism may have helped early man survive a hunt or a battle. Endorphin production is also stimulated by prolonged exercise, great excitement, severe pain, consumption of spicy foods, and orgasm. The *placebo response*, feeling better when we feel hopeful and cared for, is associated with a rise in endorphins. We know that acupuncture stimulates endorphin secretion into the spinal cord and brain, and scientists debate if it is acupuncture that triggers the placebo response, or whether the needling directly stimulates other parts of the nervous system. Acupuncture was effectively used on horses over five thousand years ago in China. Do you think horses can have a *placebo response*?

I would encourage you to engage in activities that can stimulate your body's natural production of pain blockers. Activities such as meditation, hands-on therapy, acupuncture, and aerobic exercise can complement your feelings of hopefulness to help stimulate endorphin production. So, as you can see, chronic pain may be part of your illness and diagnosis, but you don't have to be helpless in managing it.

LET ILLNESS BE A LIFE TEACHER

When Joy joins "The Ladies Who Lunch," she quickly loses her calm spirit as the women around the table question her illness and her efforts to get better. Later she concludes there is something for her to learn from her own reactions and vows to handle the situation better next time. Maybe she will face the possibility that she is angry because she still believes some of the opinions that are expressed. Maybe she wonders if she didn't somehow bring all this on herself. Perhaps she harbors an internal struggle with the question "Why me?" Joy has worked hard at learning how to manage her illness and has acknowledged that her illness is chronic, but at this time, I don't think she had fully accepted or grieved her personal losses. Joy has seen the many books that prey on the guilt of persons with chronic illness. "If you would just try (fill in the name of the miracle product, service, or practice) you will be cured!" Although Joy is a woman who has always prided herself in doing her best and she knows in her heart she has been diligent in treating her illness, the embers of self-doubt are easily ignited when the barbed insinuations from around the table suggest that her illness is due to stress, that she could get better if she tried, and that maybe she really does not want to go back to work.

Joy's anger and frustration are understandable and she lets it show, but at the end of the lunch she walks away wishing she had handled it better. She thinks if she could be more understanding, maybe they could, too.

If I can help you get in touch with your own feelings, you will gain knowledge and skill that will allow you to better manage your illness, and your life. This will allow me to be better at coaching you to increase your function, illness or not. A silver lining of learning to manage chronic illness is the opportunity to improve your general health and well-being as well.

DON'T CONFUSE MAKING PEACE WITH GIVING UP; NEVER GIVE UP

Many of my patients have done everything that was asked of them and responded to all the "should do" statements that have filled their minds, but it has come at the cost of reducing their own personal, quiet time. They feel imprisoned by their illness and are self-critical for not being able to get better. They react by working so hard at getting better they run themselves further into the ground, like the stuck car we talked about in the last section. In his book *Celebration of Discipline: The Path to Spiritual Growth*, Richard Foster describes twelve disciplines and the freedoms attained in practicing each [4]. The disciplines are categorized as Inward (mediation, prayer, fasting, study), Outward (simplicity, solitude, submission, service), and Corporate (confession, worship, guidance, celebration). He emphasizes that these activities are the means to freedom of mind and soul that will allow spiritual growth, not the end in themselves.

Mr. Foster's eighth discipline of "submission" may be particularly important for those of you who are trying to face the realities of living with illness and to make peace with it. The term submission may have a negative connotation to some, as if it means to quit trying, but Foster defines it positively as "the ability to lay down the terrible burden of always needing to get our own way" [4, p. 111]. This includes the need to fulfill all our self-prescribed expectations, day-to-day wants, and big picture life desires. Mr. Foster's freedom of submission sounds a lot like the acceptance that is required for you to move from one phase of illness to the next. Understanding this can help you avoid confusing making peace with giving up.

I have said many times that I have one of the best jobs in life, because patients teach me daily what it takes not to give up. For you, it probably starts the minute you roll out of bed. A recent patient illustrated this with her explanation of how important it was to her that she always made herself look good. Elizabeth described to me how she put on her armor every morning with each pass of the lipstick and stroke of her hair brush. She said that these actions infused her spirit with hope and commitment. It took all of her commitment on one of Seattle's recent, rare snowy days when, without a car, Elizabeth spent her morning transferring to three different buses to get to her oncologist's appointment on time. Then she walked a mile in the snow to get to my office for her second appointment of the day. By the time I saw her, the pain in her knee had become severe and needed treatment. After our appointment, she gave me the gift of allowing me to drive her home and became my first "home delivery" patient.

For those readers who are friends or family, remember that your loved one communicates how they feel through how they look. Jane was hospitalized and bed bound for over a year. A blood infection caused many of her joint replacements to become infected and her hip joints had to be removed. She couldn't walk. But every morning before I made rounds, she had her hair done and make up on. Jane had her hairdresser come to the hospital every week. One Saturday a nurse told me that Jane had canceled her usual Friday hair appointment. I knew without even seeing her that she must be feeling depressed. When I entered her room that morning, I pulled up a chair and sat down, ready to offer the encouragement and sympathy she so seldom needed or asked for.

So each morning when you prepare yourself for the day's battle of living with illness, remember it helps to put on the armor of looking your best. If you can, present your best self to the day, then gaze into the mirror, smile with self-congratulation, and commit to never giving up!

UNDERSTAND THE BUSINESS PLAN OF
AN INSURANCE COMPANY

In "Pills, Procedures, and Paperwork," Joy took action against the bureaucracy of her medical insurance company by appealing a denied claim. Her determination to build a supportive health care team paid off, as they were willing to take time to aid her efforts. By redirecting her frustration into action, she stood up for herself, resisted being discriminated against, and as a result felt more powerful.

In "Disabled, But Not Invalid," Joy is better equipped to manage these external stresses, and now must deal with the viper-like disability insurance company that turns adversarial when she makes a claim instead of paying a premium. She's already learned that persistence can pay off with her health insurer, so she is armored and ready when her disability insurer also questions her claim. After continued harassment, Joy and her husband agree that he will become legally responsible for dealing with the disability insurer, and together they begin to regain control, a step critical for both of them to cope with Joy's chronic illness. Joy receives the additional bonus of a deeper trust and increased intimacy with her husband by allowing herself to be dependent on him in this way.

The role of insurance companies acting as the general contractor for America's health care system continues to be debated. T. R. Reid in *The Healing of America* compares how health care is provided in other developed countries, such as France, Germany, Japan, the United Kingdom, Canada, as well as the United States. By the World Health Organization ratings of fairness, France is ranked 1st and the United States is 54th, out of 191 countries [5]. This low ranking is in spite of the United States spending more on health care than any other country in the world. In 2008, we spent 16% of our GDP compared to 8.1% in Japan and 9.4% in Sweden, the two healthiest countries. Then, in his chapter called "Paradox" Reid drops a bomb. He writes: "The United States is the only developed country that relies on *profit-making* health insurance companies to pay for essential and elective care" [5, p. 38]. Given this reality, Joy's experience is not so surprising.

In our clinic, we have a trained vocational and rehabilitation counselor. Like me, Don is one of the coaches for our patients and I suggest that most of them see Don to help them understand the phases of illness and learn coping strategies. When needed, Don also works with employers to develop appropriate accommodation for a chronically ill employee and to act as an advocate in a patient's claim for short- and long-term leave or disability. Most importantly, Don helps patients recapture their sense of humor when life looks bleak. He is particularly helpful during a patient's initial visits to our clinic, since it is our policy to not advocate for a patient's disability during the first six months of care. This may seem arbitrary, and we realize that policies are rules made to be broken, but our reasoning is that it is hard for a patient, and for me, to try to improve *functional ability*, while at the same time trying to prove *work disability*.

Dealing with health insurance companies, rather than disability insurers, is a different challenge. We have a full-time person in the office whose only job is to try to get our recommended treatments preauthorized by our patients' insurers. This process becomes more burdensome and costly every year, but we are lucky to have ten health care providers in the clinic to share in the burden of this cost. Small offices find this level of advocacy almost impossible, and this is where you come in. You must learn how to advocate for yourself, as Joy did. I teach patients how to write letters to their insurers. If that isn't enough I tell them to call daily and ask for the claims manager, and if that fails, ask to speak to their bosses. If that still doesn't work, I suggest they send letters to the state insurance commissioner and request the insurer speak to me directly. Why? Because, in my experience, I have never had a test or therapy denied once I was able to speak to a physician at the insurance company. This strategy works, but how do you want me to prioritize my day, on the phone with your insurer, or talking in person with you?

After you have made these efforts, and if you still have not received satisfaction from your insurer, I believe it is part of your doctor's job to do what it takes to get you the care needed. A young 23-year-old woman from eastern Washington comes to mind. Four years ago, Kayla was diagnosed with rheumatoid arthritis and had a really tough time accepting the diagnosis and the treatment. Six months ago she came to see me. After first dispelling her greatest fears (the medications would prevent her from ever having children), and helping her understand that she was still in complete control ("Kayla, I work for you!"), she got on a treatment program that made a huge difference. She opened up like a flower during her visits, even though she had to drive four hours to get to our appointments. She became so motivated she decided to begin training for a triathlon. This was something she had wanted to do for years, but she had almost given up hope it would ever be possible for her. I truly felt like her coach, and her cheerleader, as I watched her progress. But, in time, the intense swimming aggravated her shoulders joints, which, along with her wrists, had been her most damaged joints. I injected corticosteroids and continued her biologic infusion and methotrexate, but she still awoke at night with pain. She tried swimming without raising her elbows too high in order to prevent impingement, but without great improvement.

At this time, I discussed hyaluronic acid injections with her. These gel shots, originally derived from rooster comb cartilage and used for years in race horses, unfortunately were only approved for injection into the knees in humans. I reviewed the literature. There were a number of reports and controlled studies showing that these shots were also effective in the shoulder, so I asked my assistant to get them preauthorized. To my chagrin, I was told that Kayla's insurer was one of the HMOs in town, and the shots weren't covered. I asked her to connect me with a medical director at the insurer and, to my surprise, I was able to talk to a physician within a couple of days. He was interested in my proposal, and asked that I fax him the literature. Kayla got her approval and we began the series of three shots. Two months later, Kayla came in to my office beaming, "I have no pain in my shoulders and I have slept through the night."

Six months later was a proud moment for us both. She came to her appointment with a medal around her neck, her award for completing her first triathlon.

LISTEN TO YOUR BODY AND FIND YOUR OWN BALANCE

In order to have peak performance in your life, you must listen closely to your body, as well as to the advice of others. Then, you must use the knowledge you gain to change your activities and bring balance to your life. This balance is especially important in the ongoing management of your illness. For example, if you feel solely responsible for your illness, you may feel unnecessary guilt or failure if it progresses, or you do not do as well as you'd hoped. On the other hand, it is equally short-sighted to follow your doctors' recommendations to the letter, if this comes at the expense of learning to take care of yourself and finding your own means of coping.

The quiet activities that illness demands can give you the opportunity to listen to your body differently and more closely. In listening differently, you might ask whether a symptom is a new problem or a variation on a past flare. Are your fears and anxieties influencing your disease or just how you perceive it? And you need to listen to the external environment around you differently. Do you have negative people in your life that need to be tuned out? Can you pay more attention to and learn from those people who are willing to support and share with you? My experience as a physician tells me over and over again that you most likely know what you need. Which part of you—the physical, spiritual, social, emotional, or professional—needs attention today? Patients of mine who have learned to listen to what their body is telling them come to understand they cannot fix everything just by trying harder—remember the Stuck Car?

You have read how Joy learned ways to manage her illness. She learned how to ask questions and adjust those things done TO HER. For the YOU FOR YOU part of her program, Joy is learning to better manage her time, talk less, exercise as she feels able, get plenty of rest, and let go of those things she can't control. The YOU AND OTHERS part of her care program has required her to change her work, talk openly with her husband, and advocate with health and disability insurance companies. She has gained confidence and performed well in all three domains of her care program and has learned lessons that undoubtedly will help her general health as well.

I am reminded of George Burns who, on reaching the age of 90, gave sage advice on what it takes to live a long life. He said "Find a chronic illness and learn to live with it!" Joy's stories help us see how this is done.

Like Joy, you have undoubtedly had some days where you feel more optimistic, but others that, despite your best efforts, drag you down. On those hard days, an awful awareness can grab you again and again—the illness is not going to go away. These sad, difficult feelings are part of the process of *Grief and Acceptance* that characterizes the third phase of the chronic illness journey.

Phase III
Grief and Acceptance

I Cry

Today I received final approval on my disability claim. For two long years these people have constantly challenged my claim and made me the subject of their ongoing investigation. Today, they write that they have closed the books. It should be a good day, knowing this endless harassment is finally over, the security of steady income guaranteed at last, but clutching the letter I slide down the wall to the floor and weep like a child, overcome with remembering who I used to be and all the loss that is represented by this notice. It's official, I'm disabled. They believe me. Now I must also believe.

I remember the day this all began like it was yesterday. It's like a movie I often call up and replay inside my head. It was a bright day in May. My husband and I trudged up the stairs to the office of the investment firm where we both worked, he as the manager, me as a broker. I can still see myself following a few steps behind him, stoop-shouldered, each step labored and slow.

I say to his back, ashamed, "I probably won't make it a full day today. I had pain last night, didn't sleep well. Not much better this morning."

He answers softly, "We need to talk."

We go into his office, he shuts the door, and we slip seamlessly from our roles as husband and wife to employer and employee, as we have for so many years. I know the decent man sitting behind the desk has had to blur the line between manager and husband these last few years as my worsening health has resulted in more errors, more sick days, and more medical leave. I know he has been the one to cover for me. And the staff, following his lead, has covered for me too, always checking my work, hoping to catch my errors before they cost me, or the firm, or our clients any money. I have bought stock when I meant to sell, placed orders in the wrong account, written 2,000 shares on an order when I meant to write 200. If I were not who I am, the boss's wife, I probably would have been asked to resign long ago.

He looks across the desk at me and says, "Joy, it's time to hang it up."

"I'm just so tired."

"I know you are, and it's time for you to go home and rest. You're not getting any better staying on here; you're getting worse. I know you are a good broker and a responsible person, but this can't go on any longer."

"I know, but …"

"It's just a matter of time before a mistake happens that we can't fix. I support you, but you need to stop. Go home. Take care of yourself."

I cry. I cry as I leave his office. I cry as I gather my coat and briefcase. I cry all the way down the stairs and into the car and all the way home. I crawl into bed and sleep and cry and cry and sleep.

For the next several weeks, I go into the office every few days for an hour or two to say goodbye to my clients and to train the brokers and staff who will take care of them. I have hundreds of clients and we've worked together for thirteen years. I've helped them save for their retirements, prepare to send their kids to college, start companies, and buy houses. I've been to their funerals and weddings. We share trust and affection and they respond to the news of my leaving with gifts of houseplants and flowers, notes promising it won't be forever. They remind me they will be praying for me. They assure me this is temporary. I'll soon be back to work.

I cry.

Then one evening I say to my husband, "We need to talk."

We sit side by side and I stare at the floor. "We've agreed I am too ill to work," I say. "If I can't support myself anymore, I have to apply for my disability insurance."

"Why? You know I will always take care of you."

"I do know that. But, what if something happens to you? You could get sick, too. You could be killed in an accident. Then I wouldn't be safe. That's why I've been paying for this insurance all these years, to be safe. I can't wait and make the claim later, I have to make the claim now."

He cries.

In the months that follow, I no longer know who I am. I'm no longer a broker, a businesswoman, a working professional. I can no longer proudly answer the question, "What do you do?" I am just a daytime sleeper, a doctor-appointment maker, a brain-addled person filling out paperwork. Five minutes working in the garden and I collapse in pain. Twenty-minutes at the sewing machine and I am numb with fatigue. Everything I try to do is riddled with mistakes because I can't think straight. I am lost, I am no one. I am nothing.

I cry.

Months later, our firm rewards my husband for all his hard work with a trip to Hawaii. We decide that I will go along with him. A change of scene will be good for me. While he attends the morning business meetings we once went to together, I can get a massage or lie out by the pool. Who wants to get up early and go to those boring old meetings anyway? Now I can be lazy and sleep late and walk on the beach and listen to the waves and get some color in my cheeks. If I don't feel up to the evening cocktails and dinner, we just won't go. We'll get room service instead, just the two of us. It will be a fun time, a special trip.

We arrive at the hotel and make our way to the registration table to pick up our packets. His name tag says, *Senior Vice-President, Branch Office Manager*. Mine only says, *Spouse*. I fight back tears.

I turn from the table and notice people gathering to sign up for the weekend's activities. I recognize the group lining up for the tennis tournament. I know so many of those faces. The person I used to be would have been in that tennis line, with her racket under her arm, laughing and challenging the other players. The person I used to be would have played her best, maybe even won a game or two. I have been so busy being sick, I forgot about the person I used to be and how much she loved tennis. Standing in the middle of this room full of happy, smiling people, I remember her and I cry.

Today, two years later, sitting on the floor by my front door, a notice of disability approval in my hand, I am flooded again with the memories of all I once was, all that has been lost, all that these promised checks can never buy back for me. I drop my head to my knees and I cry.

Still Time

I am a gangly, long-legged, 10-year-old girl sitting on my bed in my cell-small room, hunched among pillows wedged into the corner, a book propped on my knees. The banks of casement windows that frame my bed on two sides are cranked all the way open and a warm, south Texas breeze wafts through the screens. The high hedge of Canna lilies outside my windows rustle slightly, and I stop to gaze at their wilting red, orange, and yellow blossoms and the burnt tips of their oar-shaped leaves. Summer yellow jackets fling themselves against the window screens, buzzing in frustration at the barricade that keeps them from my temperate space. The children playing yard games out in the neighborhood call to each other in muffled voices as they race from yard to unfenced yard. "Red Rover, Red Rover. Let Tommy come over!"

I have been allowed to decorate my room and chose a circus theme. My mother sewed window awnings and hung them so they make a canopy like a circus tent over my twin bed. The print fabric has jugglers in pointy hats and ladies in tutus, balanced on the backs of galloping horses. Trapeze artists fly wildly through space, arms and legs akimbo. On the wall across from the bed hangs a long shelf that displays my collection of dolls and circus animals. Below the shelf is the small desk where I do my homework.

I have just returned from my early morning swim team practice, so I feel like a rag doll, looselimbed and tired. My hair is stained acid green and smells of chlorine. I twist strands of it between my fingers and listen to the crinkling sound, like cellophane. My skin is coated white from the chlorinated pool. I lick my finger and draw a line through the film on my arm.

While I read my book, I absentmindedly peel the skin from my sunburned nose. Reading is as easy as watching a movie for me. I spend hours with Nancy Drew and the Hardy Boys, the Blue Book Biographies and every travel book our librarian recommends. Since I have already been to swim practice this morning, I know that I am liberated for the rest of the day and can read as long as I want. I will not hear the usual summer admonitions from my mother to "Do something. Go outside! Get some fresh air, get some exercise!" A long day of perfect, quiet freedom stretches out in front of me, endless and still.

I spend dozens and dozens of childhood summer afternoons just this way, quietly reading, at rest, attuned to the smallest details of the world around me. It is as if time stands still.

Then, in what seems like only moments later, I am all grown up. I get busy and get to work. I set goals and make lists and stick to schedules. I go to college and the books I must read have deadlines, tests, and term papers attached to them. I get married and have kids, and I drive them to their swim practices and diving lessons and soccer games. I fall into bed at night hoping for sweet night-time dreams; there is no room in my life for lazy daydreams. Time is linear and metered out in marching steps like the relentless ticking of a metronome. I have so many jobs to do, and fast, to keep up the pace.

Where along the way did I lose that childhood ease? Where did I lose that sense of being one with the space around me, the smallest details so vivid and clear? I remember it only dimly now, that feeling of floating weightless through the day, lofted by a hot summer breeze.

Still time. It is gone to me. I have lost it and along with it much of the most precious, private, authentic parts of myself. I have become like that trapeze artist, flying wildly through space, my arms and legs flailing.

Then I get sick and my life begins to wind down like a spinning top, wobbling at first, wandering in circles then slowing, collapsing on its side. Illness forces me to be still and I find it as hard as being imprisoned. At first, I feel locked up by illness, but over time I begin to pay attention to the world outside my bedroom window, much as I did as a child. From my bed I can hear the cows lowing in the valley below, mother calling out to calf. The sea smell rolls in from the shallow bay to the west carrying the scent of wet sand and seaweed. I rise in the morning and sit with a mug of coffee on the second story bedroom porch, a blanket draped around my shoulders. I watch the fog roll in lazily from the bay to carpet the valley like soft cotton. As the sun heats the land, the fog retreats in long ribbons, fingers beckoning—follow me, follow me. Sometimes I see an eagle glide past and count the seconds before the next slow flap of its wings and its rise on the wind. I read favorite books over again and my thoughts wander through the pages like an invited guest returning to a favorite vacation spot.

When at last I am able to rise from my bed and leave what has become the sacred, safe place of my bedroom, this sense of peace stays with me. I don't need to see people, I don't need to speak, I spend long afternoons cooking, slowly savoring the simple tasks. I clip bunches of herbs to scent the kitchen and flavor the food. There is no rush, I have all day.

In the quiet of this new life, imposed on me against my will, I once again discover still time, and find myself within it, so familiar and yet brand new.

A Gift of Grace

My grandfather thought I wasn't looking when he placed his palm over the domino tile, slowly slid it off the table and slipped it into his vest pocket. Later in the game, I saw him sneak the domino back onto the table and play it. On Sunday mornings, my grandfather quit playing dominoes for a day, slicked back his thin, gray hair, and went to his small Southern Baptist church. He put on his black robe, climbed into the pulpit and preached to a meager congregation about the wages of sin.

His long bony fingers clutched the sides of the scarred pulpit and he wagged his crooked, arthritic finger at his congregants. "Almighty God looks down from on high on all you sinners! Every one a' you deserves to be cast into the pit of hell to burn for all eternity! Y'all are teeterin' on the precipice, your sins heavy as an anvil on your back, pressing you down, down, down to the edge of the inferno. But praise be to the merciful God!"

My grandfather thrust his arm out over the podium and raised the volume a notch, "'Just before the weight a' your sins has pushed you into the flames, He has plucked you back!" He swiped at the air, pinched his thumb and forefinger together and made a sour face, as if holding a dirty, flea-bitten cat by the neck. "God is holding onta' ya' above the very pit of hell! But, sinners, there is an end to His mercy! And on that day, Almighty God will let you go, and you will plummet into the fire to burn, burn, burn! Repent! Repent now! The end is nigh!" He flung his arm over his head, palm open, empty-handed once again.

The congregation leaned forward, looked down as if to see that empty pit then looked back up at my grandfather, shaking their heads. "Amen, brother. Praise the Lord. But for the Grace of God, there go I."

I remember sitting in the front row family pew when I was too little for my feet to touch the floor, swinging my patent leather Mary Jane's back and forth as I listened to my grandfather preach. I gazed up at him doubtfully. First of all, I knew this man was a cheat at dominoes and therefore should not be trusted in any way whatsoever. Second, the kind-faced God I believed in wore a flowing white robe and sat on a big, golden throne. When I was sad or hurt, I imagined crawling into his lap for a cuddle. My God would never despise me, or fling me into the fiery pit. That was just plain silly.

I liked my father's vision of God better than my grandfather's. Daddy was a cheerful North Dakota Episcopalian and lived his life with more of a "peace that passeth understanding." His idea of God was vast, beyond our simple human ability to comprehend, so he didn't fret over it. However, he viewed the rules laid down for us as reasonable and straightforward. My father did his best to live decently, tell the truth, work hard, honor his family, and on most Sundays, go to church. When he courted my mother, his prospective father-in-law asked him if he was saved, to which my father answered with confidence, "Yes, Reverend, I have quite a little bit of money in the bank."

My father did not fear death, but he hated aging. When he hobbled down the sidewalk in his later years, bowlegged and potbellied, he would start at his reflection in a shop window and exclaim, "Who the hell is that *old* guy?" One sunny day, when he was seventy-five, my father went golfing with friends, finished the round, then fell to the ground and died in an instant from a massive heart attack. I imagined him that night, shooting through the heavens like a new born comet, on to the next adventure. I was sad I didn't get to say goodbye to my father, but for him it was the best possible death, a gift of grace.

My mother ran away from her father's house at seventeen and grew up to be a world-class Seeker of Truth. She enjoyed no peace that passeth understanding. While she did not believe the message her father preached, his words haunted her and she spent her life seeking a more comforting vision of man's relationship to God, one that would replace the frightening images hurled at her in the words from his pulpit, and in their home.

As a young girl I often accompanied my mother on her quest and witnessed the many ways believers attempt to climb into the lap of God. I saw sobbing sinners come to the altar rail to accept Christ as their personal Savior. I had my aura read and was told an aunt on the other side was going to keep my feet dancing all my life. I heard a huge choir sing praises to the Lord in glorious, jubilant harmony, accompanied by a pipe organ that was two stories high. I went to healing revivals where the crippled were felled by the awesome power of the laying on of hands and then rose and walked off the stage, leaving crutches and wheelchairs behind. I swam alongside my mother through the healing mist of a steaming hot spring; the books in our home taught me about the healing visions of Edgar Cayce and the healing foods of Adelle Davis. When I was a teen, my mother and her friends often gathered on their knees around our living room coffee table and spoke in tongues. This, they told me, was the language of the angels.

Mother discovered many truths, both new and old, on her journey and she stitched them together to make her own comforting crazy quilt of faith. She came to believe we all arrived on Earth with lessons to learn, and when we mastered them we would be sent to the next planet to learn the next, higher lesson. In her later years, she held a conviction there were aliens inhabiting our planet, available to serve as our spiritual guides. She climbed a California mountain hoping to meet up with them, but she did not find them there on that day.

I think my mother thoroughly enjoyed her restless life with its series of grace-filled moments, but it seemed to me she never stopped running. She would find one truth, embrace it for a year or two and then move to the next. In an endless series, she ran away from one view of the absolute truth just as eagerly as she ran toward the next. The exhausting tension of that journey never stilled in her. The expectation of punishment and the shame of not being good enough made its way into every chapter of her life.

When she learned she had leukemia at 72, her first question was, "What did I do wrong to be punished in this way?"

I did some meandering of my own as I grew up, as might be expected of a child brought up in a family of such disparate beliefs. I sang in the choir at our Episcopal church and went to church camp every summer. I joined many youth groups—Methodist Youth Fellowship, Presbyteens and even Baptist Training Union. I had a Jewish boyfriend who took me to his sister's bat mitzvah and a Mormon boyfriend who asked me to wait while he served his mission. I did not wait, but went on to college and majored in literature. I had to study every major philosophical movement of the last two centuries, from the Puritans to the transcendentalists, from the pragmatists to the idealists. Each of these, and many others, shaped my view of the world and my view of the nature and behavior of love, both human and divine.

In time, my searching wound down and I found an easy peace and faith within myself, more mystical than my father's, but less desperate than my mother's. Although I no longer went to any church, there were two scriptures from my Bible reading days that continued to inform my faith. One was: This is the day which the Lord hath made, we will be glad and rejoice in it [6]. The other: All things work together for good to them that love God [7]. I have tried to seek the joy in every day and I believe there is a possible good outcome to everything that happens in life.

A few years after I got sick I traveled back home to care for my mother. She had been diagnosed with acute leukemia and I knew she had little time left. She did not believe this and at first even questioned the accuracy of the diagnosis. For a time, she searched for a cure outside the boundaries of modern science, but finally submitted to chemotherapy treatment. Allowing her doctor to inject what she considered to be poison into her body went against every fiber in her being and made her sick in body and in spirit. Afterward, she enjoyed a brief remission, but refused a second round of chemotherapy.

I asked her to say out loud to me what she understood this refusal of treatment to mean. With tears streaming down her face, she said, "It means I would rather die than endure another round of chemotherapy." At these words, we held each other and cried together in a terrible release of grief and acceptance.

On the last day of my mother's life, she was struggling hard with her passage, perhaps revisited by the ghosts of her father and his predictions of what might await her on the other side. I climbed on the bed with her to comfort her. I sang *Amazing Grace* softly into her ear over and over, only I changed the words. I could imagine her God reaching out for her on that long, hard day, but I believed he would see her as I did, as a *gem*, not a *wretch*.

After mother died, I went home and emerged from my grief thinking about the life I had in front of me, rather than the one just completed. I pulled my dusty copy of the *New International Bible Dictionary* from the shelf and looked up *grace* [8]. I needed to understand what this strange concept really meant. The illnesses I had were not expected to kill me, as my parents' illnesses had, but in a very real sense illness had taken my life away. I was sentenced to live with physical pain, in real time, indefinitely. I could not work. I could not even plan my days. I could not expect to be cured. Going forward, how was I to rejoice in each day? How could long-term illness work for my good? Maybe this idea of grace could help me.

I learned from the dictionary that *grace*, or the *gift of grace*, is variously defined. In one sense, it is "that which affords joy, pleasure, delight, charm, sweetness and loveliness." This sounded wonderful; I'd love to wrap myself in those feelings, layered like a shawl over the hurt. It is also compared to "the kindness of a Master to a Slave, thereby by analogy, the kindness of God to man, or the favor bestowed upon sinners through Jesus Christ." This was less appealing, as it sounded more like my granddaddy. According to Christian law, grace is the "medium or influence enabling the believer to persevere in the spiritual life" and is associated with various "gifts of the spirit; such as knowing, thanksgiving or gratitude."

So, I thought, here is the core of it. Grace does not just initiate faith; it sustains faith, even in the hardest times. It is a gift that allows us to be grateful for what is, rather than mourn what is no longer. It is an active way of living, rather than a passive way of believing. To live with grace means to live exactly as those two favorite scriptures instructed—appreciate each day and look for the good in it. Further, grace is especially available to the humble, which I was glad to read, as illness had surely been humbling for me.

I next pulled down *Bartlett's Familiar Quotations*, and read references to grace which included this song from the 1500s [9]:

> *My mind to me a kingdom is;*
> *Such perfect joy therein I find,*
> *As far exceeds all earthly bliss*
> *That God and Nature hath assigned.*
> *Though much I want that most would have,*
> *Yet still my mind forbids to crave.*
> *My mind to me an empire is,*
> *While grace affordeth health.*

The song describes a life that is not dependent on earthly pleasures or possessions, a life in which there is no longing. Attaining this state, the song tells us, brings health. But as in the song *Amazing Grace*, the reference is to spiritual, rather than literal, physical health.

Grace is a solace, not a cure.

I searched further. In her book, *Walking on Water: Reflections on Faith and Art*, Madeline L'Engle quotes Aeschylus, the father of Greek tragedy, as he defines the grace given to those in pain [10]:

> *In our sleep, pain that cannot forget*
> *falls drop by drop upon the heart*
> *and in our own despair,*
> *against our will, comes wisdom*
> *through the awful grace of God.*

The wise man tells us grace does not take away the pain or suffering, but affords wisdom in spite of it. It is not a gift that we must seek, but one that is channeled to us through our own despair. Even against our will, this awful grace will come to us as a gift from God.

I began to look at my new life through this ancient lens and in time came to realize that my illness did offer me a special opportunity for an enriched spiritual life, one that had not been so easily accessible when I was healthy. I've been physically forced to slow down and as I've submitted to this new way of living, the coil of rage and frustration at being sick has slowly unwound, those roiling feelings replaced with a calm center. From that center, I can now see that even my illness has worked for my good. I have ample time to notice and rejoice in each day, only with more appreciation for the single, present moment than ever before. In the stillness and quiet that illness demands, I have come to feel more connected, rather than less, to the vast universe I inhabit. I feel more like I am part of an organic, pulsing whole and less like I am alone and striving.

As I have been sidelined from the busy world of personal ambition and drive that I used to occupy, I have become more empathic, and less judgmental. I more easily see the worth in others and realize there can be many right answers to life's questions. I've learned to accept the value of those who are different from me and I've also learned to accept the value in the person I have become. I can see the worthy purpose in the life I now live.

It is a rich irony to learn that there is a special peace to be found in the journey through suffering. Because of this revelation, I have come to see myself not as a sick person, but as a person who enjoys a life that is full and abundant. I see myself as a healthy person with an illness. To live fully and to be healthy, even while sick, is the great mystery and blessing that has come with my illness. It is my gift of grace. And even if I do get physically well someday, I don't think this gift will be taken from me, for it is who I am now. Like the innocent child I used to be, through grace, I am privileged each day to sit on the lap of God.

Dr. Overman on Grief and Acceptance: The Waves of Loss

The experience of grief and acceptance is not unique to dealing with illness; these are universal life experiences. Cultures and religious traditions have evolved in different ways to help us handle this shared human experience. In the Jewish faith, mourning for lost loved ones is highly ritualized and lasts one year, while in the Baha'i tradition there are no mourning rituals. Buddhists say prayers weekly for 49 days, with the first week being the most important, while Catholic friends and family share in funeral masses and other celebrations.

What rituals can we access to manage the recurring experience of loss that occurs with chronic illness? Whether you lose an activity, the dignity of independence, or a future dream, these are not easily shared or even perceived by your friends and family and these unexpected moments of awareness and grief are harder to build rituals around. As you read Joy's stories, you were invited to join in one person's experience of *Grief and Acceptance*. Each of us can learn from her experience and each of us can teach others of our own, as my patients have generously taught me.

Each time Joy acknowledges what she has lost and the tears well up in her eyes, it is as if she is walking down the beach and a wave unexpectedly splashes her, soaking her feet. The water recedes, but as she continues her walk, the waves return again and again to splash her. A big wave hits Joy and brings tears while she is standing in a hotel lobby and is suddenly reminded of how she used to be able to play tennis. Another comes when she finally receives the insurance approval she fought so hard to win. Chronically ill patients may become better over time at navigating the waves of loss, but the surges will continue to occur, often when least expected. As with the illness itself, the recurring feelings of loss and grief are also chronic and not likely to ever go away completely.

When you feel like Joy did, what can you do to survive the waves of grief that nearly drown you? How do you positively emerge from the realization that you will never again be the person you once were and that your life will now be different from what you planned?

In his book *Different Seasons*, Rev. Dale Turner addresses a common question asked by those who face the feelings of crisis and frustration associated with getting sick and being sick: "Why me?" [11]. Don't we all ask this question? If, when the recurring waves of grief overwhelm you, your response is to ask this question over and over, how can you ever break the cycle of self-pity? My advice is to pick a different metaphor. When the undertow is just about to take you under, stop struggling, roll over, float and see if the next wave might take you back to the security of dry land. Rev. Turner reminds us of one way we can roll over and look up when grief's undertow pulls us under—he suggests we merely change our perspective and ask the question differently. Instead of asking "Why me?" ask "Why am I so lucky?" Don't take this wrong, he isn't suggesting that your loss and grief is a good thing, but he does affirm that we all have blessings that may be obscured by our sorrows and therefore aren't acknowledged. These may be the small things—a smile, a cloud, a phone call, or a reflection about days past. Asking the question differently can help us see beauty in each moment. Moving from grief to Living Well requires this ongoing change in perspective. Start now.

Start investing in your passions and simple joys, and soon you will be able to navigate the big waves and the undertow.

RECOGNIZE THE ROGUE WAVE

The waves of grief may surprise you at the most unexpected times, even as you enjoy a pleasant walk down the beach, your feet sinking into the wet sand. Sometimes, as was the case with my patient Craig, the wave can knock you down completely and only after struggling back onto your feet do you recognize what happened.

Today, Craig is my superstar patient, but at our first visit Craig was suicidal, completely overwhelmed with physical pain, the loss of his job, and a future that seemed hopeless. Craig suffered an injury while at work at the Department of Labor and Industry. Together, we fought through his crisis and the frustration he endured in his dealings with the claims managers. Over many months he worked hard to regain his former upbeat self, fighting through his pain to slowly build an exercise program that helped him let go of his anger. With each victory I felt happy for Craig and proud of how well he found answers drawn from the experiences of his past. Sure, he implemented many suggestions that I offered him, but it was the confidence he regained in himself and his own solutions that really propelled him forward. Each month I enjoyed walking into my office for our appointment just to see his smile and hear his update.

I remember as if it were yesterday one particular morning when I entered Craig's room excited to be his cheerleader, as always. This time I saw Craig's face, head askew and eyes looking down, and I felt like my own energy was being drained into what I could instantly see was a black hole of despair.

A rogue wave had washed over Craig and turned him upside down, and neither of us understood what had happened or what to do. I was overcome with an ominous feeling. I didn't know what to do for him. But then I thought of the work I was doing with the phases of chronic illness. I told Craig I had an idea about what might be going on. I suggested that he had been hit with a wave of grief, and that even though he was building a positive life today, perhaps he had not yet really accepted that he would never go back to being the old Craig again.

Craig put his face in his hands and I could see tears dripping to the floor between his fingers. Craig was experiencing a very real grief at the death of his former self.

How would you feel if you got an A on every assignment in a class and received an F for your final grade? Craig had done everything asked of him, utilized everything he learned from his past and performed beautifully. For Craig, a passing grade meant returning to his former self. Now he felt betrayed and lost as he realized he wasn't going to pass the course as he envisioned. He now knew that returning to his former self was never going to happen.

After minutes of silence, Craig looked at me and I couldn't find the words to comfort him, so I gave him a hug. Even in the shared sorrow of this moment, I had a deep sense of awareness that Craig had just taken a necessary step toward reconstructing a new life of *Living Well* with his illness.

TAKE TIME TO CRY AND ACKNOWLEDGE YOUR LOSSES

Like Craig, Joy reached the point when she was forced to accept that her illness and its impacts would not go away; that she had a chronic illness. In "I Cry," Joy tells of the time she finally realizes she is really sick, must quit her job, and is stripped of her work identity. Even though she is in a supportive marriage, she feels alone as she deals with her experience. Her feelings of loss and despair come and go, and like her symptoms, their timing and intensity are unpredictable. Where are you?

I trust that by now you have overcome the misconception that, "There's nothing to be done." You've pulled yourself out of crisis and learned to manage the impacts on the physical, emotional, social, and spiritual aspects of your life. Even still, perhaps you've held on to the hope that this is all temporary, in the end your illness will go away. Now you may be starting to understand that it won't.

This is the most difficult phase to "doctor." There are no pills or words that heal grief. I have previously described the different aspects of the doctor–patient relationship. In the beginning, you needed hope and my role as a physician was to offer it to you through listening, diagnosing, acknowledging, and treating. The healing properties of touch are found in many traditional medical practices along with the use of symbolic dress and props. During those early visits, wearing my white coat, using my stethoscope, and my laying on of hands may be powerful comforts. As you stabilized, I became more of a coach, teaching you about illness, therapies, self-care, and healing, while never giving up my search for new ways to treat your disease. But during your grief our relationship is a true partnership since I have no special expertise in navigating one of life's great challenges—helping you, or any patient, find acceptance.

Recently I saw a patient, Joanne, who plays the organ for a very large church in Seattle. As luck would have it, before we even met, I accepted a referral from the Arthritis Foundation to give a talk at her church's final Health Education class of the fall. She helped me market the class, which deepened our relationship and increased my desire to help her. I was trying to get her ready for the demands of a busy Christmas season that included four services each Sunday, filled with her holiday organ music, but I was challenged by the pain of her arthritis and her sense of despair. The first shot I gave her did not help. I used ultrasound to better see where she had joint swelling and the second shot seemed to hit the spot, but I could tell she still wasn't feeling well. However, at her next visit I sensed a change. Joanne became animated as she described what had transpired. Yes, her wrist no longer bothered her, but that seemed incidental, she told me. I had referred her to our counselor and it was this meeting that had been so helpful.

"I let go of my expectations," she said, "especially regarding my family."

She later shared with me that she had struggled under the life-long criticism of her nearly 80-year-old father. Sadly, the buoyancy she felt that day proved to be short-lived, as he continued to be critical of her. I learned from her experience that it is particularly important to understand it takes many, many successful *letting go* efforts to change the internal wiring of self-doubt associated with past trauma. If you can remember how you felt when the load of criticism was lifted from your shoulders the first time and continue *letting go*, slowly the old wiring will change and the external trigger won't keep activating your self-doubt.

While there is a case to be made that some stress can be beneficial and even healthy for us, the gap between our expectations and our perceived ability to achieve those expectations would fall under what I define as *bad stress*. To lessen this kind of stress, we need to either change our expectations or improve our ability to manage it. How confident are you that you can change someone else's behavior? What expectations do you have for your partner, parents, children, co-workers, or friends? Can you affect their actions, or do you need to think about doing what Joanne did? To let go is to take an important step toward acceptance.

A physician acquaintance of mine, Dr. Bill Gruber, accidentally acquired hepatitis C during his surgical career. He wrote a book about his experience titled *Letting Go: A Memoir*, in which he shares his journey to find himself after he was forced to quit medicine and accept a life that was no longer defined by being a doctor. His doctoring to a patient who had rheumatoid arthritis, and for whom he had performed many surgeries, led him out of his darkness, but not in the way you might guess. His patient, Mark Smetko, moved to the east coast after an accident, which meant he could no longer work as a train engineer, the joy of his life. The two continued to communicate through letters. While Dr. Gruber initially helped Mark deal with the loss of his life's passion and build a new life, in time their friendship expanded and their physician–patient relationship seemed to reverse. They shared stories about baseball and railroads and doctoring—of passion, accomplishments, and near misses. Mark, the engineer, showed Bill, the doctor, how to heal, and then how to find joy and meaning outside of medicine, just as he had left behind the clank of the tracks and the shrill whistle of the engine. They cared for each other and they shared letting go.

Joanne let go of relationships she couldn't control; Dr. Bill let go of a self-image built around his work. Both had to let go to find peace.

FIND YOUR PLACE OF PEACE

Joy's mood takes a turn when in "Still Time" she remembers a peaceful childhood day. Adulthood, with its pressures and responsibilities, has been distracting and consuming, but illness has forced her to stop and reflect. Out of the memories of her youth, Joy finds *Still Time*, the antidote to the *Snake in the Mist*. Many of my patients tell me how they have found their own place of peace. Some have happy childhood memories; some have a dream world. Some find peace in their faith, in nature, or in listening to music. Others spend time chanting, meditating, singing, painting, exercising, visualizing, all in order to capture a peaceful calm within the dark mist.

My patients bring me wonderful stories about activities that helped them find their way out of the mist. Gladys, an 82-year-old patient of mine, gave me a beautifully framed calligraphy that still hangs on my office wall. It says:

Remember yesterday
Live today
Cherish tomorrow

I had been treating Gladys for fatigue and depression for a year. During our office visits she often spoke of her despondency and the loss of her will to live despite many trials of antidepressant medications. One day she mentioned she used to paint with watercolors. I prodded her to paint a picture for me, but on the next visit Gladys brought me no picture and no change in her outlook. It was the same for many following visits, but I kept prodding her. Then, one day, I could tell she was different the moment I saw her face. I noticed she was holding a sack and after our introductory comments and update, she told me she had something to show me.

Out of her sack came watercolor paintings—not one or two, but ten or fifteen, all of a scene looking through a window of a favorite cottage she had not visited for five years, since her husband passed away. Although the setting was the same, each scene was different—children playing on the beach, sunrise, sunset, and stormy days were depicted in soft, confluent colors. Gladys had clearly found again her place of peace and painting was what helped her get there. Once again she could remember yesterday, live today, and cherish tomorrow, which included her grandchildren and her great-grandchildren.

I have one of Gladys's pictures on the wall and it reminds me that there are pathways into a person's soul that medications sometimes cannot reach. Through her painting, Gladys found a way to quiet her mind, open her heart, and bring meaning to her life again. This was critical for her and is critical for all who travel with illness. It is another light that can lead us through the difficult trials of *Grief and Acceptance*, and bring *Living Well* into sight.

TAKE CONTROL OF YOUR OWN WELL-BEING

The following is a checklist of questions I give patients as they stabilize and start to feel more hopeful. It is important to go back through these questions during every phase. To pass through grief and on to acceptance, you will again need to consider each of these questions. The list identifies dimensions of self-awareness that are important to coping, managing, and living well with your chronic illness.

ILLNESS MANAGEMENT—HOW ARE YOU DOING?

- **Orienting**—Where are you: in crisis? learning to cope? grieving? living well?
- **Coping**—Are you depressed? confident? angry? optimistic? fearful?
- **Understanding**—What do you think causes and keeps your illness going?

- **Coaching**—Who or what helps you build confidence in managing your care?
- **Monitoring**—Do you know what medicines you take? why? how much? the effects?
- **Eating**—How does your diet affect you? Do you have food sensitivities?
- **Preventing flares and re-injuries**—Do you practice pacing, proper movement and stress management?
- **Exercising and function**—What is your program? How do your goals change day to day?
- **Sleeping**—Is it restful? Do you snore or have restless legs? Why do you lie awake?
- **Managing your pain**—Do you have a pain management program that works for you?
- **Touching**—Your body needs it. Are you giving and receiving it?
- **Relaxing**—How do you prevent and relieve stress and distress?
- **Support and caring**—How do you get what you need? Is it enough?
- **Solving problems**—What are your legal, financial, family, or disability issues?
- **Living**—Have you changed the gifts you share? What is your next creative opportunity?
- **Meaning**—What meaning does your illness have for you?

How are you doing in each of the areas above? I believe there is synergy in being balanced and achieving small improvements in all areas, rather than overdoing it in a few. What goals for each dimension might you write down for yourself? What functional improvements would you like to accomplish as a result of address-ing these questions? Does trying to achieve fixed goals stress you more, or move you toward living well? It is important that you not make any activity your sole goal or an unachievable destina-tion because increased stress will be your only reward. I advise you to recognize how each one works with the others, then you allow improvement to occur naturally, leaving the "should do's" out of it.

DISCOVER THE GIFT OF GRACE

One of my patients, Susie, gave me a little book with quotes and reminders. She loved the story of Dorothy in *The Wizard of Oz*. Dorothy had lost hope that she could ever go home again, and watched in despair as her last chance to leave Oz, the hot air balloon, drifted away into the sky. But then, Glinda the Good Witch told Dorothy that the power to go home had always been hers. All she had to do was click her heels together three times. Dorothy clicked, and home she went.

Susie allowed Dorothy to be a symbol of the power she had within her to find grace. This was not easy for a 30-year-old who spent as many days in the hospital as out during the last year of her life. However, each day she found ways to be upbeat, to smile, to say thank you, and to care—even when life was difficult. She liked to kid me about being too serious and she quoted passages from *The Tao of Pooh*.

When Suzie approached what she knew was the end of her life, she experienced the ultimate grace. At this time, she clicked her heels and set limits on her treatment. Joy's reflection was also true for Susie, "Grace is a solace, not a cure."

Phase IV
Living Well

Joy's Top Ten List for Living Well, Even While Sick

1. Take care of yourself first.
2. Never, never, never give up.
3. Learn to be honest about how you are feeling.
4. Enroll in the School of Whatever Works.
5. Make friends with fatigue.
6. Live as a child.
7. Step out of the box.
8. Search for silver linings.
9. Find a way to share your gifts.
10. Be still.

My list of the top ten ways to live well, even while sick, evolved over many years. It has been reviewed and refined countless times as I have experimented and tested what works for me and for my unique conditions. For example, in the first edition of *You Don't LOOK Sick*, number 1 on the list was: Put yourself first. I decided that this is too simple and reads as a little selfish. So now number 1 is: Take care of yourself first. This allows for the assumption that, even in illness, we want and need to care for others. I caution myself that I can't do this unless I am realistic about my own needs within the complex reality of chronic illness.

Number 10 on the list used to be: Never take any medicine that will make you fat. Here I was alluding to the fact that even though there is much you can't control in your illness, you can and should have some say over things that really matter to you. Whether you must endure the side effects of a given medication can be an area of compromise and discussion with your physician. Maybe for some bad breath or a decreased interest in sex represents an intolerable side effect, and will prompt a request of your physician for another choice. For me, the intolerable side effect is weight gain. Out on the speaker's circuit, this rule got me into nothing but trouble. Many patients must take steroids, for example, and for me to say they have a choice to do otherwise, in spite of weight gain, was to treat a serious issue too lightly. That item has been replaced with something more useful and, I hope, universal: Be still.

Your list might, and probably should, be different from mine, but the process of making such a list is valuable. It keeps your focus on what does work, rather than what doesn't. It keeps you looking for the positives in your life and reminds you to reward success. It holds you accountable to apply what you have learned. It allows you to mature in this journey and demonstrate that maturity. Most of the principles on my list have been touched on in the stories Dr. Overman and I have written, but here I expound on the ten special ones that have lasted and continue to support me in my journey. I encourage you to begin your own Top Ten List for living well, even while sick.

TAKE CARE OF YOURSELF FIRST

I was brought up in southern Texas in the 1950s. I was taught, as were most women of that generation and region that someday I would grow up to take care of a family. In preparation for this role, by the time I was 9 years old I was doing all the laundry and ironing for my two older brothers and also cleaning the bathroom that we shared. My brothers and my father had their chores, too, but it is interesting to note that none of their duties involved cleaning up the messes made by the women in the household.

Later, in 1980, when I was going through a divorce, my husband told our marriage counselor that he felt I had failed to meet his personal needs. I objected to this, saying that since I had a full time job and the additional income I earned was essential to our family's support, I was meeting many needs and had done the best I could. He remained firm in his opinion that the demands of my job were no excuse for my failure to meet his personal needs. This was, to him, my role, regardless. I remember a friend saying to me later, "Most husbands are fine with their wives working, as long it doesn't require them to change at all."

His opinion about the role of a wife was not at all unusual for that time, and in strong marriages spouses do honor a desire to try to meet the needs of their loved one. But a lot has changed since those early days when women were just beginning to enjoy meaningful careers and face the conflicts that came with that. Cultural change has required married couples to seek ways to balance independence, opportunity, and family, and, in the intervening years, American men have stepped up to take on more duties related to household and family. Still, I think that many women continue to place a higher priority on meeting the needs of others and therefore carry a greater burden.

Today, many hard-working mothers hang on to the notion that they can, and should, be able to do it all—manage a promising career, maintain a loving marriage, and raise thriving children. A recent study at the University of Washington compared women who work outside the home to stay-at-home mothers. They found working women to be generally happier and reported that the stimulation of challenges outside the home do have real benefits. However, when looking at a third category, the women who held on to the belief that they had to do it all, they found this group was more susceptible to depression than either working women or stay-at-home mothers. Put another way, women who accept life's limitations have less depression [12].

More women than men get chronic autoimmune diseases. Part of this probably has to do with our complex and cyclical hormonal systems, but I'd submit part of it might also be related to our tendency to take better care of everyone else than we take care of ourselves.

My husband, Dan, was a single father for five years before we married. All three of his teenage children lived with him during that time. He once observed to me, "I have learned I must take care of myself first. If I don't I am no good to anyone else." After we married, I had this wonderful relationship to nurture, a demanding career, and six children to bring up in our combined family. The thought of putting my own needs first seemed impossible. However, I was reminded that he had been a single, working parent like me and had been faced with the same demands, and this lesson was what he took away from the experience. I have tried to follow his advice. Now, when I get in a muddle, I ask myself three questions:

1. *What is really going on here?*
   The answer is not what I'd like, or what I think should be, or what I fantasize, but rather the result of taking an honest look at present circumstances that are making me feel stressed and uncomfortable.
2. *What do I need to say or do to take loving care of myself?*
   The operative word here is *loving* care. In this situation, am I treating myself and my needs with the kindness and consideration I would be willing to offer others?
3. *What is my power for the good?*
   This third question is the most important of all because if I can't see that I have any power for the good, I'd be wise to remove myself from the situation entirely.

I find that taking the time to consider and answer these questions helps bring me clarity and relieves avoidable stress.

NEVER, NEVER, NEVER GIVE UP

One evening Dan and I went to dinner with a couple who wanted to discuss how we were managing our life together since I had become ill. They told us they were having a hard time adjusting to the husband's recent diagnosis of rheumatoid arthritis.

He was in considerable pain and, as a pianist, his life was sadly compromised, but he was resistant to accept either the diagnosis or the treatment offered. He wanted to try some alternative therapies and he wanted to be able to tell his wife how he was feeling each day in a way that would allow her to be more receptive and sympathetic. She, on the other hand, wanted to *hear less* about how her husband was feeling and *do more* about it. They both had good points and we had a lively discussion.

After our dinner conversation my husband summarized with an insightful comment, "When Joy became sick the most important thing she did for *me* was to never give up pursuing answers as to what was wrong with her and what to do about it. The most important thing I did for *Joy* was to listen to what she found out." It was my job to find my own answers; it was his to lend support and a sympathetic ear.

A friend of mine made this comment after reading about the long process I went through to win an insurance claim appeal for chiropractic treatment. He said, "This seems like a lot of work for $600. Will your readers find the effort worth it?" To me, the victory had little to do with the amount of money or even the amount of time involved to win the claim; it had to do with never giving up when I felt I was in the right. It had to do with taking care of myself and demanding fair treatment. There is little about feeling sick all or most of the time that lends a sense of power. Never giving up in my pursuit of accurate information, respectful professional treatment, personal growth and spiritual peace makes me feel empowered, and therefore healthier.

A commitment to never give up doesn't only involve advocacy and a demand for fair treatment. It also involves staying informed about new research, therapies, and treatments that offer continuing hope that improvement is possible. It is a balancing act to make peace with the current understanding that your illness will not go away, and at the same time, hold out hope that your health and function can improve over time. Living well with illness requires that we do both. There are so many fine organizations dedicated to helping the chronically ill, it's hard to list them all, but part of any illness management plan should be to seek out those patient advocacy and research groups relevant to your symptoms, get on their mailing lists, attend their conferences if possible, and keep abreast of advances in knowledge and treatment that may help improve your function and quality of life. Our Resource section can help you get started.

LEARN TO BE HONEST ABOUT HOW YOU ARE FEELING

One of the many daily challenges of living with chronic illness is how to answer the simple question, "How are you?" The polite answer is, "Fine, thanks." Much of the time I am not fine, but I was taught by my parents I should not complain or, even worse, whine. Illness has taught me that telling the truth about how I am feeling is important to being an authentic person, even if it is not a happy statement. I have also learned that if this news is not laden with emotion, fear, or self-pity, most people react with kindness.

One warm and sunny spring day I attended a committee meeting of an organization that I serve. We decided to meet outdoors and had spread a blanket under a tree; one member even brought lemonade. It should have been a lovely gathering, but I was in the midst of a hellish, painful flare that had been going on for weeks and had dragged myself to the meeting only because I was the committee chair. I found myself unable to follow, much less lead, the discussion. I was distracted by pain, muted by medication, and groggy with fatigue. Sitting on the hard ground was making it worse. Finally I said, "I think most of you know I have a chronic illness, and I'm having a really bad day, so please be patient with me. I'm doing the best I can."

The supportive response was immediate; one person volunteered to take over some of my tasks and another began to take meeting notes. Afterward, a former physician who was on the committee told me he would like to talk further with me about invisible illness; not because he was a doctor, but because he also had a chronic illness. Knowing this allowed us to forge a more meaningful friendship and he gave me helpful feedback on this book.

Later, I took a two-week symposium on writing narrative nonfiction. I was uncomfortable revealing to the group on the very first day that I had a chronic illness and was writing about it. I just don't like to define myself as a sick person, especially to strangers, and I thought I would be diminished in their eyes. Instead, at the end of the first meeting my classmates swarmed around me with questions about my condition. One woman, crippled by childhood polio, approached me with her walker and said, "Oh, I just love medical stories!"

As time has passed, and after many experiences like these, the discomfort I used to feel in talking about my illness has faded. Now that I've made peace with my illness, it is not laden with all the emotion I felt in the early *Getting Sick* years. I'm not as defensive about being believed, either. Now, telling someone I have a chronic illness carries no more emotional weight for me than telling someone I wear glasses. It's just part of who I am. The question I must answer these days is "What does this person need to know?" For example, if I am taking on a new volunteer responsibility, I need to share the reality of my limitations with those who will depend on me. If I make a new friend, at some point I want to share with this person why I don't take phone calls during my afternoon rest, or why I may be less available than other friends because my illness demands that I spend a lot of time alone and quiet. In other situations, like a casual friendship or a brief exchange at a party, my illness is not relevant. If I sense I am speaking with a person who is judgmental or insensitive, it is not in my interest to fuel their negativity. This process of getting comfortable with telling, and with not telling, has been freeing.

When we moved to Austin, we settled in a small, friendly neighborhood. I knew my neighbors would find out about my illness in time, but I didn't want to explain it over and over, one person at a time. I was tired of talking about being sick by then. My solution was to tell the person in the neighborhood who always knew what was going on and kept everyone up to date. She took care of telling others for me. The people who were to become my good friends came to me and asked for more detail.

ENROLL IN THE SCHOOL OF WHATEVER WORKS

One of the comments I hear over and over is, "I told my doctor I had symptom A and he gave me drug B. I tried it for a week and it didn't work. He doesn't know what he is doing." I find this attitude sad and troubling. The patient expects the doctor to know everything, fire a magic bullet, and hit the bull's-eye on the first shot. If this first try is a miss, the patient holds the doctor entirely responsible for making a mistake. The menu of doctors is vast, but it is miniscule compared to the variety and combinations and dosages of medications available to treat any given symptom or set of symptoms. Then there is the precision of patient reporting that, if not an art, is at least a learned skill. To say a doctor doesn't know what he or she is doing after reporting one symptom, trying one treatment, at one dose, for one week, is not only an unfair and ill-informed position, it can be a dangerous one.

The assumption that the whole universe of alternative or traditional medicine is quackery is equally troubling. Most have histories far longer than our Western practices. Discovering the treatments, of which Western medicine is one, that resonate with my particular temperament and condition has been time well spent, and I do not find the alternative therapies that are helpful to me to be incompatible with Western medicine.

I have a policy to have one doctor in the role of team leader, or as Dr. Overman would say, head coach. While I lived in Washington State, Dr. Overman knew every practitioner I was seeing, every therapy I was doing, and all medications or supplements I was taking to manage my illness. He was my gatekeeper and all other providers were asked to copy him on tests and treatments. I do the same with the new team of doctors I have in Austin.

I also have a policy to not deal with any Western, alternative, or traditional practitioners who express a rigid, negative bias against their peers on the other side of the aisle. Dr. Overman made sense to me when he said, "I'm a rheumatologist, frequently the physician of last resort. I treat the illnesses that lie in the gray areas of medicine; those with vague symptoms, unclear causes, and unknown cures. If I don't have the answer to your problem, I will work with any trained practitioner who will share information with me and perhaps help you in ways that I can't."

As time goes by, symptoms change and so will effective treatment. About seven years after I was diagnosed, I went into remission from my interstitial cystitis and no longer took any medication. Several years later, my symptoms returned. The drug

I am taking today did not exist when I was first diagnosed, and it is more effective than anything I tried previously. Getting from A, onset of symptoms, to B, current treatment available, to C, remission, and finally to D, finding a new, effective treatment, is a natural, logical and even predictable process in dealing with long-term illness. It is never over. There is always something new to learn and things constantly shift and change. There is no graduation date from the School of Whatever Works.

MAKE FRIENDS WITH FATIGUE

I struggle with fatigue and have been forced to assess and rank what drains my energy in ways I never contemplated before. Some activities are simply no longer within my capabilities, like playing tennis, but others I can still enjoy, like a limited social life and the opportunity to be a community volunteer. I have learned my best energy is between ten in the morning and two in the afternoon. By the late afternoon I am fatigued. I know that for me, rest requires being prone for several hours, with my mind and my voice as silent as possible. Then there is my nighttime social life. What can I still do? What should I avoid? Why?

I love to entertain, especially to have friends over for dinner. I love the menu planning, shopping, table setting, a day of cooking and the lingering conversation by the fire over coffee and dessert. Now I find that at some time after I set the table, but before I welcome the guests, my energy tank is already hovering at E. I just can't enjoy the process the way I used to because it requires a larger store of energy than I possess in a single day. If I want to have guests for dinner now, I must approach it differently. I need to spread the effort over several days, so things that can be done earlier, like the shopping, table setting, and some prep are handled before the day of the event. I choose simpler menus and my husband has taken on some of the cooking. We have ice cream and berries instead of a fancy dessert. I also schedule an hour or two in the late afternoon to rest in bed, before the guests arrive. By making these adjustments and managing the day better, I can still find the strength to do something I love. More often these days, instead of having friends over for dinner, we meet in restaurants.

I feel best on the days when I write quietly early in the morning and rest in bed for several hours later in the afternoon. There are exceptions, of course, but this is my habit and it works for me. When my husband and I travel with friends, we tell them that while we look forward to going out with them and exploring during the day I need to be back by about three in the afternoon for my rest period. Otherwise, I won't be able to enjoy the evening.

Invariably, our friends say, "Oh, goody, rest period! Do we get to have rest period, too?" I've learned that rest period is something we all miss from kindergarten, including the little snack we enjoyed while we took our rest. I remember graham crackers and orange juice at my school, now I have a few crackers and some cheese. My friends respect this time by not calling me between three and five in the afternoon and tell me they are jealous that I get to have a rest period every day. I keep telling them that they can take a rest period, too. They don't have to get sick first!

One of the things I often hear when I speak at patient conferences is the difficulty patients have in slowing down. People seem to feel if they don't do all they used to, the illness will have beaten them. They will have given in to illness, or given up on getting well. Even though they recognize their symptoms are worse when they are overactive or stressed, they forge on, determined the illness will not control them. At one meeting recently, in the midst of a question-and-answer period about the importance of rest, a patient in the audience broke down and cried as she tried to describe how hard it was for her to slow down. Like so many others, she saw her illness as an enemy and something she had to keep fighting against, or else the illness would win. I tried to tell her the illness was part of herself, not a separate thing and not her enemy. I said, "If you will just give this resting thing a chance, I guarantee, you are going to love it!" I can testify that I'm so glad I made friends with fatigue.

LIVE AS A CHILD

Young children are a lot like puppies. They wake up, roll around happily for a little while, get tired, and instantly drop to the floor and sleep until they are ready for the next round. Kids live completely in the present moment. They don't use up their energy trying to impress people. They don't hold grudges; if they're mad they get it out and get it over with. They freely show their affection, and also love to be held and hugged and tucked in at night. They insist upon their independence when possible, and allow themselves to be taken care of when necessary.

The best example I know for living as a child was my friend Charles. I got to know Charles after he read the first edition of *You Don't LOOK Sick* and contacted me to see if I'd meet with him to talk about the ideas in the book. He had endured a brain injury and extensive surgery, but he continued to suffer seizures and was confronted with the uncertainty and reality of long-term illness. When we first met for lunch, Charles was facing a very difficult decision. His company had offered him long-term disability, but to agree to the contract meant he had to give up his work identity and accept that he would never go back to the career he so loved. I could sympathize with this terrible time of grief and acceptance, as I had gone through this myself years before. We laughed that day as I tried to convince him that since he had disability insurance, this illness meant he would get paid for *not* working. This wasn't the very worst thing that could ever happen to him in his whole life.

Charles and I ended up on the same theater board and became dear friends, meeting for lunch every few months for the next eight years. We always talked about illness and health and how to live well, no matter how life presented itself. After Charles went on disability, he faced more challenges. He needed to move from a house into a condo and he had to make a thousand decisions about the move. This was stressful and overtaxing to his brain. He later had to accept that the unpredictability of his seizures meant he should no longer drive a car.

Even as all this was going on, Charles was learning how to live as a child. He took unabashed delight in discovering downtown living and making new friends in the high rise he called his "vertical neighborhood." He became the social chairman for the building and organized a monthly cocktail party, a dinner club and frequent events. He bought a hot little sports car that he wasn't supposed to drive, but he figured other people would love to drive it—even if it meant having Charles along as the bossy passenger riding shotgun. He continued to enjoy the arts and supported the arts throughout the city, on boards, in the audience, as an advocate and donor. He was endlessly available to friends to talk, go to parties, have dinner, and just enjoy living.

At one of our lunches he told me he'd discovered a way to keep from being so preoccupied with his illness, a challenge we all face. Charles bought four sets of weekly plastic pill minders, the kind with four cubicles for each day of the week labeled Morning, Noon, Eve and Bedtime. He popped open all the lids and perched on his bed with his myriad bottles of medications. He said it took him a very long time to fill all one hundred and twelve cubicles with his prescribed doses. When he was finished, he slapped the bed and announced, "There, I don't have to think about that for another whole month!"

In recent years, Charles's seizures increased in frequency and severity, but his joy in living each day, treasuring the moment and relishing his friendships increased right along with his symptoms. He made several trips to Europe, even traveling alone for a few days, just to prove he could do it. He had a friend he agreed to call at the end of each day to report where he was, that he was okay, and that he had not had a seizure in a strange country. When we met for lunch he always picked the restaurant, as he knew them all. He walked me around and introduced me to the owners, waiters, hostesses, and chefs. When we finally sat down and I asked how he was doing, he just said, "Great!" Then he launched into telling me about the new restaurant, or friend, or recent trip that he enjoyed. Illness was still there, and real, and operating in the background, but Charles seemed to have transcended it in favor of relishing each precious, present moment. He seemed to glow from within at the delight of experiencing every bit of joy and vibrancy in his life.

Charles died in early 2012. He'd been out for the evening with friends, feeling fine. At about one in the morning, he returned home and fixed himself a bowl of ice cream. He was found the next morning lying on the floor of his kitchen, ice cream on the counter, freezer still open. I went to see him at the hospital to say goodbye. He was on life support, pending the arrival of the dear friend who held his medical power of attorney. He had decided to be an organ donor, of course, so these preparations were also being made. While he was living so fully and joyously, he had taken time to be realistic about what might happen next and he had planned everything just so.

I sat in the waiting room for a few hours with his friends from his downtown condo building. They were grief stricken. They'd only just met Charles; he was their social chair, the jolly one, the one who was there for everyone. How could the place survive without his bright light and smiling face?

I told them how Charles and I met, how brave he had been in facing his illness and building a new life that some might see as painfully diminished. I told them how we had lunch every few months for many years to talk about illness, and health, and trying to live fully no matter what the circumstances. I said he had used his brain injury as a platform upon which to build a life that expressed his essence: kind, good-humored, generous, and more than anything—available.

These friends, who had only known Charles a short time, turned to me and said, "Brain injury, what brain injury? We didn't know he had a brain injury." They never knew Charles as anyone but the wonderful person he became, more of what he essentially was, the boy in the man, filled with wonder and delight in each day he had left. Now, *that* is living as a child.

STEP OUT OF THE BOX

Once or twice a year I take on something that is out of my range, something that is too much for me, and will probably make me sick if I can accomplish it at all. I do this because I yearn to feel more alive. I also do it on the chance that I've gotten better and don't know it. I simply can't live well, while sick, unless I step out of my little sick box once in a while. This thinking has helped me to avoid experiencing illness as a prison that I am trapped within. I know my illness is not static and I do have choices about how I live with it. If I think an activity or adventure is worth the price I may pay for overextending myself, I have the power to make this choice. Earlier I wrote about patients who push and strive every day beyond the boundaries of their illnesses. This exhausting and futile effort is ineffective and can even be damaging to the long-term management of their health, but the occasional, intentional stretching of the boundaries of illness, done with preparation and foresight is another choice entirely.

I stepped out of the box when I played the part of Jenny Malone in Neil Simon's *Chapter Two*, but I learned to safely and successfully use narcotics for pain during the run of the play. I went on a cruise with my husband, which I thought would be a big step out of the box, but it turned out cruising was a great way for me to travel. I only had to pack and unpack once, I chose only the activities I felt well enough to do, and I was able to go to our cabin to rest whenever I needed to. I will do more of this kind of stepping out if I can.

This ongoing book project has been a big step out of the box, and has led to the opportunity to speak to chronically ill patients all over the country. These short trips to patient conferences require careful management of my time and energy, and I am usually exhausted by the time I return home. They are certainly a step out of the box, but they are deeply meaningful to me personally and have often given me the chance to work with Dr. Overman again. We hope they offer worthwhile support to those with whom we share our message.

Later in this *Living Well* section, I share a story about stepping out of the box to travel alone to my high school reunion, an experience that had its consequences, but was worth it in the end.

When I shared my theory about stepping out of the box with Dr. Overman, he commented, "Not only do you test the boundaries of your illness, but you give yourself something to look forward to." Perhaps that's the point.

SEARCH FOR SILVER LININGS

My mother told me it was wrong ever to use my illness as an excuse, because then I might come to like it, and then I might not want it to go away. As with so many other comments I have heard, this one could only be made by someone who has never had a chronic illness. To me there ought to be some advantages to being sick, such as permission to say, "Gee, I'm so sorry I can't come to the birthday party for your 5-year-old with thirty rowdy, screaming kids, but I just don't feel well enough." Or, "I would love to join your weekly four-hour, mean-spirited Hearts game, but my illness doesn't allow me to sit in a straight-backed chair for that long." What's wrong with that? To me, that's a silver lining.

I haven't had a single cold in well over a decade and I've only had the flu once. I figure my immune system is so over-active, none of the little bugs are able to survive in my body long enough to take hold. Of course, I often feel sick, and have endured wretched seasonal allergies, but no seasonal colds or flu. I am very proud about this. When flu season arrives I like to tell everyone, "Oh, I don't need to get a shot; I don't get the flu." I love to hug and kiss people who are sniffling and sneezing and when they say, "Oh, don't touch me; I have a terrible cold," I brag about my immunity and I am gleefully obnoxious. This is another silver lining!

One of the sad consequences of divorce is that it can erode one's ability to trust. We don't go into a marriage thinking it could ever fail, but if it does we are understandably wary of making that same mistake again. Even after I married happily for the second time, I found myself waiting for the marriage to get into trouble. When I became ill, I could not take care of myself. I could not work to support myself, and I was completely vulnerable. Why would this man stay with me, I thought, I am of no use. Despite my fears, I was not betrayed or abandoned, but rather I was offered my husband's complete support. As a result I was able to fall into a deep well of trust and love with him that was beyond anything I'd ever known before. I don't know if we would have found this depth of trust had I not become sick and put both of us in a position to experience the strength and breadth of our love through this shared struggle.

I remember when my mother became ill and I needed to go stay with her and care for her. I remained with her for the planned two weeks, but it wasn't enough. She needed more time from me. I was afraid to tell my husband. I thought he would be mad and feel neglected if I didn't come home as planned. I feared I would have to choose between her needs and his. When I did call and tell him I felt I should stay longer, I confessed that I feared losing him if I didn't put him first. There was an old tape still playing in my head from the past, and I feared he might leave me. His reply was, "Where would I go? I'm already home. I'll wait here for you—take care of your mother." This was a lovely silver lining, maybe the best so far.

FIND A WAY TO SHARE YOUR GIFTS

For the first months, or even years, after finding a name for my illness, every available brain cell and every ounce of energy I had was needed to determine what to do about it. However, the time came when my illness had stabilized somewhat and I understood it was not going to go away, or kill me, at least not any time soon. I realized I needed to find a way to focus on more than just me, my illness, and how I was feeling each day. I had become too self-absorbed and too preoccupied with illness. The only solution was to find something to do that wasn't about me, to share my gifts, such as they were now.

First I accepted a position on the board of a community foundation, an organization that exists to support broad community needs. The foundation was young, had no paid staff, and was really just getting started in establishing practices and procedures. Up to this time, no one on the twelve-member board had the time, or the inclination, to address the laborious task of creating a tracking system and entering all the historical data about donors and grants since the inception of the foundation. The fact that my illness required me to spend a lot of time at home and in bed allowed me to spend several months on this task. I'd crawl into bed with my computer each day, pull out some records and work through entering them, refining and improving the record keeping system as I went along. I eventually became chair of the foundation and when I resigned three years later, the board gave me a going away gift, a letterbox from Tiffany's. In the lid was a plaque inscribed with the sweetest possible sentiment, "Your gifts keep on giving."

Later I was invited to join a theater board. I served on various committees and again, I could work on projects some board members, with their full-time careers and young families, might find too time consuming. I became president of that board and also serve other groups in the city. As I look back at these years of volunteering, speaking about our book, learning more about the arts, education and philanthropy, I see that I am the one who has received a gift. I have collected valuable and useful skills. I've gained new knowledge and new friends. I did not expect that learning to give my new gifts in a new way would, in the end, be such a great gift to me.

BE STILL

Recently, a friend asked me to lunch to meet the mother of a teenage girl who had been diagnosed with chronic fatigue syndrome. The situation was tragic; this vital young woman could no longer attend school each day. She could no longer play sports and didn't know if she would be well enough to go to college. The mother was desperately seeking answers, even flying with her daughter to another state to seek the best possible treatment. She was determined to find avenues to help her daughter, doing everything she could think of to do. I thought she was heroic and her daughter was incredibly fortunate to have such a strong and determined advocate.

At some point in our conversation, I heard myself say something that surprised me. Do you know that feeling? That you never knew you believed something until it came out of your mouth. The mother was focused on diagnoses, treatment, therapies, studies, and causes and this is what we had been discussing intently throughout our lunch. I reached out and touched her shoulder.

She stopped talking, and I said, "You know, if your daughter can embrace the reality of this illness in her life and make peace with it, she will have the opportunity to learn, at a very young age, what most of us never learn in our whole lives. She can learn to be still. Help her do that and you will have given her a very great gift."

Later I thought about our conversation and how illness has changed my life in two very big ways. One consequence is that I did not get to do all I had planned to do with my life. The other is that I learned to be still. At this point, I have to say that the second of those two consequences has been the most meaningful and the most life altering. I am grateful now that I was forced by illness to learn this. It is in the stillness and quiet that I have learned to feel most at peace, most whole, most healthy, and most connected to the vast, miraculous universe that surrounds me. Before, when I was so healthy and had so much to do, I didn't have time for this. Now, I cannot imagine who I would be without it.

Stepping Out of the Box

Now that I've entered the *Living Well* phase of chronic illness, I must say I've become quite skilled at heeding the boundaries set by my activity monitor. This is the built-in system that alerts me when I am risking a flare-up of my symptoms because I've been too active or stressed. Now when the alarm goes off, as if on autopilot, I climb into bed as soon as I can and rest until the pain subsides and my energy tank refills a little. I also know how to be preemptive about activity. I've learned to take the time to rest even when I'm not experiencing the warning signs of symptoms, or take special care to rest before I take on an activity that I know will be draining for me. The good news is I have learned to maximize my function and stability, minimize my pain and fatigue and do so with less medication. The bad news is I feel like I have narrowed my life down to two basic activities each day, shopping for dinner and preparing dinner. My husband thinks this is a positive aspect of my illness, as I have become a much better cook, but I don't feel like I'm good at much of anything else. I think it's time for me to take a step out of the little sick box I'm living in, stretch my wings, and test those boundaries. I want to see what more I can do. Who knows? Maybe I am doing better than I realize. Heck, maybe I got well along the way and failed to notice.

While immersed in these thoughts, I receive a flyer in the mail announcing an upcoming high school reunion. The reunion committee has planned a three-day weekend on the Texas gulf coast island where many of us spent our spring breaks and summer vacations. Next I receive an e-mail from a classmate inviting me to stay at her beach cottage for the reunion weekend. She is asking only a group of nine women, no men allowed. Oh, how I'd love to go! But, I haven't traveled without my husband for years. I'm afraid of lifting things, or getting too tired. I might have a flare of pain, disabling fatigue, or a bad case of brain fog or, God forbid, all of the above, all at once. It would be an awfully big step out of the box for me to travel alone to this event filled with social demands, take care of all my own things, and manage my own schedule. But, what am I thinking? This is just the opportunity I've been seeking. I decide to make the trip. After all, it's not going to kill me.

I make the trip to the coast without any problems and join the other guests at the cottage. We head down to the beach for a walk, but after just a few hundred yards, my dreaded activity monitor starts to beep. It's already been a long, grueling day and I know I need to stop and rest. Sadly, I head back to the cottage, turning to watch my friends as they grow smaller in the distance. I can hear their soft laughter and I resent not being with them. I feel left out. Maybe I shouldn't have come.

The next day we spend a lazy morning in our pajamas, with unkempt hair and no make-up and drink pots of coffee. We have gathered here from states across the country, as well as many cities scattered across Texas. One by one, we tell our life stories, braiding our separate adult lives into the childhoods that we shared long before I got sick. I feel like I am back in the fold, a part of a collective experience. Today I am not just cooking dinner; I am not just being a crummy old sick person. Like my classmates, I have my own accomplishments to share. I've been to college, had two careers and two kids and my own lousy divorce. I've been broke and started over, and met the right guy and raised our six combined kids. I've become an author. The last few years, I've been so busy with doctors appointments and the dictates of my activity monitor, I've pushed all that aside. Today, I can see that being sick is the short, small part of my whole, long life and I'm so glad I came.

Tonight could be trouble. Tonight, we all go to the open-air pavilion at the island's ferry landing for a Mexican dinner and dancing to a live band. I am zinging with excitement and anticipation—and apprehension. It is sultry and steamy here on the beach. My hair has curled into a damp cap, and I put on a T-shirt and silky print coveralls. The class assembles for a panoramic photo on the pavilion bleachers. I'm down near the front, flanked by old friends. I turn around to look at all the still-familiar faces, many now with thinning hair and wrinkles around the eyes. I can't wait to catch up with everyone. I'm really, really glad I came.

After we get our dinner and drinks, small groups perch on concrete picnic tables to renew acquaintances. Women linger in the rest room telling tales. We smoke forbidden cigarettes, like we used to do behind the gym. Then we start to dance. How long has it been since I danced? I love to dance. I go out on the floor, the music beats on and I dance and dance and dance with all the boys who never asked me out in high school. Then a line starts to form and, gathering our classmates as we go, we snake around the pavilion until we make a big circle on the dance floor. Couples are pushed to the center one by one, and we clap and yell at them to "Walk the Dog," to do the "Sloop" and the "Stroll," the "Gator" and the "Texas Two-Step." If you aren't from the South, these names may carry no meaning, but they are mean measures of dancing, I can tell you.

Then the band rolls into its signature number, "Shout!" The whole class is on the floor, bobbing to the beat, arms and voices raised, transported back to that innocent, hopeful time before we had our paunchy bellies and crow's feet. Finally the cops come and shut the party down, just like the old days.

Our group of women returns to the cottage and we settle on the back porch that faces the white dunes of the beach. We talk late into the night, gazing out at the rows of small, glistening waves, lit by the moon as they crest. Finally we go to bed and keep each other awake, sharing memories. I think this might be the most fun I have ever had in my whole life.

When I wake up the next morning, I linger in bed, reviewing the evening and gradually I realize something strange has happened. Somewhere between the class photo and the wave watching, my activity monitor must have broken. I know I vastly exceeded my boundaries, but the alarm completely failed to alert me. Even more shocking, I can't remember having any pain, any fatigue, or even any brain fog. How did I do that? What happened?

Then I remember my disability insurer and their relentless claim that I am a fraud and someday they will prove it. Maybe they were right all along. Maybe all this time I've been malingering. If last night is any measure, clearly I am not physically sick at all. Maybe I am mentally ill. Maybe I wasn't ever really sick; maybe I'm just a slacker. I feel so ashamed.

I get up, dress, and pack to leave the coast. There is a farewell brunch at a café down on the wharf before we board the car ferry to the mainland. I spend the night with a friend in San Antonio and go to bed late, again. Now I am looking forward to getting back home. I am also beginning to feel the weight of my excesses of the last few days. It's like I've been on a teeter-totter, enjoying the view and stuck at a sky-high level of wellness, but now I can feel the balance shift as I begin to drift back to Earth. I will land with a thud.

The next morning, I prepare to catch a flight to the West coast where I will meet my husband for a few days of rest. Confident the flight leaves at 10 AM, I get up and dress, put my last items into my bag, glance at my ticket and only then see that my flight leaves at 9! How could I have been so sure, so wrong? Why didn't I check the ticket? I don't have a direct flight and I have to make a connection with only an hour and a half layover. I frantically call the airline and reserve a seat for the next flight. My friend drives me to the airport and I check in. As I hurry down the jet way, I begin to feel it, the familiar pain coming on, starting low in the pelvis, wrapping around my hips, creeping up my back. I don't dare take anything strong for the pain right now; I have too many responsibilities and no one to help me.

I make it on to the flight. The worsening pain is exacerbated as I lift my bag into the overhead bin and belt myself into the small airline seat. We land and I have just enough time to make my connection. I hurry to the gate and check in again, by now bleary-eyed with fatigue and stooped over with pain. I see I have enough time to go to the restroom, so I leave the waiting area and then return to wearily await the boarding call. When I hear the announcement, I queue up with the other passengers, board and hoist my bag once again into the overhead bin and buckle in. I wish I could just lie down in the aisle.

Then a man presents himself at my side and insists the seat I have taken belongs to him. The flight attendant checks my boarding pass and says in alarm, "I don't know how we missed this. This is not your flight; yours is at the next gate." She looked at her watch, "It was due to leave five minutes ago."

I scramble for my things, my heart pounding. The pain alarm is shrieking a red alert. I make it to the other gate just as they are about to lock the door, but they let me on and have not given away my seat. What happened? I checked in, I got my boarding pass, everything was in order. Then I realize that when I went to restroom I must have returned to gate 4B, not 4A. How could I do such a thing? How could I have missed the gigantic sign hanging above the reception area? Why didn't I note the flight number or listen to the announcement?

Of course, the dreaded brain fog. I'm slogging through this hellish day in a quagmire of brain fog. My worst fear has been realized; I have brain fog, numbing fatigue, and debilitating pain all at once—and I'm all alone.

As we lift off the tarmac and head west toward the strong embrace of my waiting husband, I can finally take a pain pill. I tilt the seat back and close my eyes. I feel grateful for the last-minute shards of luck and grace that got me safely to this last leg of my big adventure. I am aware that this grace, as always, is undeserved.

When I get home I will take a few days rest, and probably a few more days of pain medication. I know that eventually, the teeter-totter that is my life with illness will find balance on its fulcrum once again. I will make a few nice dinners. I'll pull out my reunion pictures and savor every one. I'll have time to reflect and I know I will be so very, very glad I took this chance to step out of the box. It may take a while, but in another year or so I'll muster up my courage and strength and I'll do it again.

I have since learned that my experience of enjoying a temporary surge of well-being is not an uncommon phenomenon. It seems that people who are sick, when completely engaged in a beloved activity, can briefly transcend their symptoms. I don't know how it works; perhaps a huge wash of pleasure endorphins overwhelms the illness, or maybe the mind is so completely engaged it briefly forgets about being sick. I know a dose of strong narcotic pain medication can temporarily reduce symptoms and even the remembrance of them, but it often comes with mental dullness and a drunken clumsiness. My reunion phenomenon, which I have experienced a few more times since that magical night, admittedly came with a couple of really good, cold margaritas, but I had no sense of being drunk, or muted, and with all that dancing, certainly not clumsy. So I regard these brief episodes of freedom from pain and illness as a mysterious gift. It's not like grace, this stepping out of the box. These times represent a gift that I consciously give myself. It is a gift that I have earned, by learning to manage my illness, and a gift that will cost me, for breaking my own rules. Still, it is a gift.

Natural High

I have completed the final drafts of the stories I have written for this book. Now I am edgy and restless without the discipline of daily writing, and so I have returned to work on my next project, a novel. It is the story of Celia Gene Williamson, a young, small-town girl with the gift of second sight. CeeGee, as she is called, is able to tell what the future holds for other people, but not for herself. With the help of a wise old man who expounds on life as he sits on his front porch tapping his cane and rocking his chair against creaky wooden floorboards, she slowly learns what her gift really means. "You have not been given a gift," her old friend teaches her, "you have a gift to give. It is not for you, it's for the others."

My young character learns that when she foretells the future, it is not always good news and therefore will not always be well received. She will find that the information she shares may be used wisely or not, exactly as the recipient chooses. Most importantly, she will learn that when she tells someone the direction they are headed, she offers that person the opportunity to change direction, and thereby change the future. The future is not cast in stone, but evolves, subject to many forces beyond her special gift. I guess it is no surprise that I am drawn to a story about how life does not always turn out the way we planned and the various ways a gift can be given.

What my young character learns about giving her gift in part reflects the strange paradox that is at the heart of every writer's life. A writer engages in a process that in the beginning is intensely personal and private, but in the end must become public and laid open to any manner of scrutiny and judgment. Once out in the world, the work no longer belongs to the author, but to the reader. Completing this process requires an emotional surrender, not unlike the one I made as a young mother, watching my first born child, a baby only yesterday, marching bravely down the sidewalk to the school bus.

Tonight, as I sit on my porch in the spring dusk, waiting for night to surround me, I ponder gifts, the ones I have received from this long project and the ones I hope it might offer when, once again, it becomes yours, not mine.

From where I sit, I can see the swallows have returned to build their home on top of our wind chime. At first, my husband thought he could control where the little birds would nest. Each year when he saw the swallows were back, making their muddy nest of dirt and twigs, he hauled out the hose and sprayed off the top of the wind chime, then turned it on their berry-filled droppings on the concrete below. The little birds flapped their wings furiously, circling round and round until he went indoors, then immediately began re-building the nest and dropping their berry stains. The next day my husband would hose again; then the swallows would build again; hose again; build again. Now I see them in the yard chasing the larger birds away from the half-finished nest on top of the wind chime that is their annual home, as it has been for the last few years. We finally learned that we could not chase the swallows away, and if we could, we would have more bugs in the summer. Thanks to their stubborn persistence and huge appetites, we don't.

A robin red breast hops across the grass and I stay very still as I watch him lean over, peck at the ground and actually pop back up with a fat worm wriggling in his beak. It's as if an illustration I've seen in dozens of children's books has materialized before my eyes in real time. I am amazed; I have never before witnessed this.

A young buck wanders up from the creek adjacent to our property. Alerted to my presence by his animal radar, he raises a handsome, newly antlered head, notes my location, and gazes at me for several minutes, seeming to gauge his risk. Then, unperturbed, he drops his head and delicately raises a hind leg to scratch behind his ear, which flops forward over his face like the untrimmed bangs of a teenager.

Here in the deepening shadows are the referents to what I have learned through the experience of writing about illness. I have found that sometimes the best thing to do is to just sit back and let nature take its course. I try to live my life without futilely fighting battles I cannot win. I've realized that what seems bad at first might turn out later to be good, and in ways I never anticipated. I have learned to be very still, and within that stillness pay close attention. Sometimes in the small quiet I experience important new things.

I've become so comfortable with the principles I've written about on these pages, and I live so fully within the boundaries of my small world. I am more even shocked when I venture out and hear how differently other people view illness and what to do about it.

I have noticed there seems to be a growing devotion to alternative or traditional practices of healing and with it a growing suspicion of Western medicine. I stood in a dinner buffet line next to a woman who had fancy elastic support bandages wrapped around both her hands and wrists. When I inquired what had happened to her she told me she had osteoarthritis in her hands and when they ached, immobilizing them with the bandages seemed to help. Good idea, I thought. I wish I could do that; wrap myself up with bandages, shoulder to hip. Then, in a rapid series of statements, she went on to tell me her doctor had advised her against activities that were destroying what remained of her thumb joints, but she was determined to ignore her doctor's advice. That's just not me, she stated with pride. When I mentioned the arthritis drug I was finding so beneficial, she said yes, she had tried it once, for a day, got a headache, and decided she couldn't take "that kind of stuff." She didn't believe in drugs.

Then she told me her daughter had a chronic illness. She wished her daughter would submit to a very gentle form of bodywork, which she knew would provide the cure for her, as it had for many others with diseases that Western doctors could not cure. She ticked off an amazing list of unrelated health problems she was certain could be cured with this practice. When I asked the name of this miracle treatment, she repeated it was a very gentle form of bodywork. She also felt her daughter needed to look at why she had *drawn illness to herself.*

At this point, I gripped the sides of my dinner plate and vowed not to engage in a battle I could not win. I reminded myself her experience was not my experience, and so I should not judge. I decided I would not ask where she bought her bandages. I really missed my mother, who shared some of this woman's mindset, but remained a generous and loving spirit. My mother's beliefs ran contrary to conventional wisdom, but they expanded her vision. She did not become smug in an absolute certainty, nor did she harshly judge others.

My buffet companion embraced the same kind of rigidity in her opinions as those who are convinced only drugs and surgery can cure what ails them, and that bodywork is a thinly veiled form of prostitution. Saddest of all she blamed her daughter—both for being sick and for not getting well. This was heartbreaking to me.

Dr. Overman and I have spent years now traveling and speaking about the messages of this book and the phases of chronic illness. We've benefited from a lot of valuable feedback. Some patients say they found in me an ally, a person like themselves, with the same struggles and questions and sorrows about illness. They have said that after reading our book they feel less alone, as we hoped. Dr. Overman has helped readers assess what to expect from their physicians, and encouraged them to be the best patient they can be. They say they now understand health care is a shared responsibility.

Readers have said there needs to be an exposé about disability insurers and their unethical treatment of clients like me. Before they read our book, they thought only the insurers were being cheated. They had seen those grainy videos of people who claimed injury, but were caught flinging heavy objects into the backs of pickup trucks, then jumping agilely on big Harleys bought with their dirty insurance money. Now, they are paying closer attention to the sponsors of those newscasts and recognize there is more than one side to this issue.

We've heard hundreds of unique, personal stories of the trials of learning to cope with long-term illness and what patients find to be the most challenging aspects. Americans are proud of being able to figure out how to fix everything. This makes it hard to accept those conditions which cannot presently be fixed. Sometimes our culture reacts to this by not believing the condition exists at all, or by laying blame on the victim. Patients seem to struggle most with making peace with an illness, living within its boundaries and learning to be still. And yet, this challenge is precisely the path to living well with illness. We hope this second edition of our book can continue to offer a roadmap and guideposts to help others on their way. We know our stories are not our reader's stories, that each reader will come to this book with their own set of experiences, offering the opportunity for learning and growth. We only hope our stories encourage openness to this process.

Before I go, I want to conclude with good news: I am feeling much better than I did when we first began this book. I don't know why exactly, because I've tried just about every treatment known to man, including gentle bodywork. It's sometimes hard to tell which among the many offerings have been beneficial. Oddly, if I think it is a drug therapy that is helping me, I become a sort of reverse addict and am eager to go off the medication that has caused me to feel better. I want so much to believe it's *me* that's better, not the drug that has made me better.

But I truly believe, at least in part, that it is the stories we have shared with you and with each other that have made me better. I, too, have found recognition and support from our readers and audiences who have been willing to share their stories with me. Writing these stories, hearing yours, and working with Dr. Overman and others has given me a forum to look at my life and how I live it. Speaking aloud about my beliefs has required me to become conscious in my choices, and held me to a responsibility to practice what I preach. I have had a chance to review my long history with illness and find in it a teacher. Knowing that people who are like me will read our book and perhaps relate to our experiences and struggles has made me feel less alone. I thank you. I hope the future is good for you, full and meaningful.

Share your gifts.

Dr. Overman on Living Well:
Weaving the Web of Wellness

There wasn't a course when I was in medical school called, *Living Well*, but today there are all kinds of wellness and longevity clinics that have cropped up around the country. There are lists of alternative therapies that promise wellness—from supplements to energy therapies, from mineral springs to Bikram, a hot room yoga. Each of these practices offer ways to engender *wellness*, but they do not address living well *with* illness. Phase four, *Living Well*, is less about a destination called wellness and more about the process of living. It is no longer about what we do to our bodies, rather how our spirit can thrive in spite of our bodies. What does illness have to teach you about *Living Well*? Let me start with my own story.

Some time ago, after a CT scan, I was diagnosed with coronary atherosclerosis. The report indicated my condition was worse than 90% of men my age. With this news my cardiac illness journey began; I subsequently developed recurrent episodes of atrial fibrillation requiring electric shock treatments and medical therapy. I want to share only a few snapshots from these past ten years, not Joy's big screen movie, but hopefully enough to help you see how this book has had personal meaning for me as well.

Not long after the CT scan, I was having a stressful day in the office. I ate my lunch, hurriedly and on the run, so I wouldn't be late for my first afternoon patient. Then suddenly, I felt a burning in my chest, which in the past I would have diagnosed as typical heartburn. Now, given the results of the CT scan, the symptoms could mean something different. I wondered if this was heart pain known as angina. I tried to think logically and stay calm. What should I do? I talked to a partner. I checked my pulse and felt some skipped beats. I jokingly told my nurse to resuscitate me if I dropped to the floor. However, my repressed fear was distracting. I saw two or three more patients, and then had an EKG. When I read it, it appeared to be okay, but there was increased voltage. Such a change is a possible complication of high blood pressure, but an athletic heart can look the same. I tried to breathe slowly and relax, but my mind was flooded with indecision and clinical self-doubt. I could hear the common medical school saying in my mind, "He who has himself for a physician, has a fool for a physician."

It was then that I remembered the story of the stuck car and realized I had driven off the road, and was unknowingly pushing on the accelerator and starting to spin my wheels. I forced myself to breathe more easily and over the afternoon my symptoms passed. Eventually, I had other tests that were reassuring, though I was now aware that there would be new challenges to come and phases to navigate. During that one afternoon, the crisis of *Getting Sick* began. I experienced anxiety, fear and the feeling of being confined in the box of getting sick so many of you have been through. All of the sudden I could not see my future. I was lost in the mist. I knew I would have to part the mist, come face to face with the snake, and then learn to live well. I have now personally experienced various coping strategies and have cycled through the illness phases we have explored together.

I developed atrial fibrillation for the first time after drinking ice water during a long afternoon bike ride. I wasn't sure what was going on and tried to cycle on. Ultimately, I had to call my wife to pick me up, and she later confessed that I looked dead lying on the side of the road awaiting her arrival. I have been in the hospital twice and the ER five times. Each time has been a learning experience. I have realized that living well 80% of the time is not enough. I had to try to learn to listen to my own music and dance my own dance in order to find the ways to live well.

First, I had set the goal of exercising more regularly, though less intensively, but my schedule always seemed to get in the way. Then I moved my practice north of Seattle, nine miles away from my home. Sitting in my car in the freeway rush hour parking lot one evening, I realized how I could help myself in two ways. Since that time I have been a bicycle commuter. First, I now exercise a minimum of an hour and a half per day when I would have been just sitting in my car in traffic. And second, according to my environmentalist son who calculated the annual CO_2 savings, I will save the planet about 3.8 tons of carbon dioxide from car exhaust.

I spent some time with a colleague social worker who also teaches meditation. I had some prior experience, but always had trouble keeping my mind from wandering. Len said, "Steve, you will never be able to sit still; you need bicycle meditation." The light bulb went on. I understood that instead of focusing on my breathing or relaxing from the tip of my toes to my scalp, I could calm my mind by being aware of each pedal stroke, my upper body posture, and shoulder relaxation. I learned to do this for at least half the trip, then I would let my mind go to the problems of the day. Other times I practice what is called *passage* meditation. I learned this from a patient who referred me to www.easwaran. org [13]. Eknath Easwaran was a professor of English literature in India before he came to the United States on a Fulbright exchange program. He stayed on in this country to become the originator of passage meditation and in 1961 he began the Blue Mountain Center of Meditation. Below his picture on their website is the quote, "By virtue of being human, each of us has the capacity to choose, to change, to grow." The daily email I get from the center, which is nondenominational, gives me a chance to step back and look at current challenges differently. This has become part of my morning ritual after riding my bike to work, doing a little gym workout and sitting down for my cup of coffee. There have been other steps in my learning to live well, but now let's get back to you.

I hope you have gotten out of the ditch, but have you slipped back into *Getting Sick*? Are you still working on driving differently? Joy had to learn to travel at a different pace, and with help she taught herself to enjoy the new scenery and destinations. Have you changed expectations? How have you progressed through *Being Sick* and *Grief and Acceptance*? Are you listening differently and learning a lot? I know there is so much to learn—new medicines, insurance programs, symptom management and diet and exercise programs. You may have found other helpful resources: how-to guidebooks like *The Chronic Illness Workbook: Strategies and Solutions for Taking Back Your Life* by Patricia Fennell [1]. This book can help you move through the phases with workbook exercises. Another workbook by a well-known researcher and educator is *Living a Healthy Life with Chronic Conditions*, which is a text used in group education programs developed by Kate Lorig, Ph.D. [16]. *How to Be Sick: A Buddhist-Inspired Guide for the Chronically Ill and Their Caregivers* [17] was written by Toni Bernhard, a former law professor who became ill in her prime. In it she explains how Buddhist principles helped her cope with limited energy and solitude. For the special challenges facing younger adult patients, *Life Disrupted: Getting Real about Chronic Illness in Your Twenties and Thirties*, by Laurie Edwards, may offer practical advice [18]. She addresses the financial downside of chronic illness, and gives useful tips on how to stay in the workforce despite chronic illness.

You may have reached out to friends and family and found a support group, either for your illness or just your general well-being. If not, the list of foundations and patient support associations in our Resources may be helpful to you. I hope you have assembled your own health care team and found just the right coach for you. With all of these tools, you are on your way to weaving your own web of wellness. The following tips may also help.

WEAVE YOUR OWN WEB OF WELLNESS

Earlier I mentioned my patient, Susie, and the little booklet of quotes and reminders that she gave me for my birthday. Susie shared some of her favorite life lessons at the beginning of the booklet, taped a penny from the year I was born inside the front cover, and instructed me to fill in the remaining pages. Susie's first selection was from the *Tao of Pooh*. It said, "The surest way to become tense, awkward and confused is to develop a mind that tries too hard—one that thinks too much. The animals in the Forest don't think too much; they just ARE. But with people ... it's a case of 'I think, therefore I am confused'" [19].

Sadly, Susie died from her illness. Thinking of those we have lost, like Susie and Joy's friend Charles, helps remind us of what we loved about them, and how our actions today honor their memory and what we learned from them. Susie loved to kid me about thinking too much, and trying too hard. Though she was a graduate researcher and understood the value of science, she knew it was her friends, family, and church that helped her to live well. My brother Mark played spoons and laughed hilariously. My father, Jesse, loved to play jokes on his brothers and used to tell me to TT—Think Tall. I cared deeply about each of these people, and each died slowly after a chronic decline. Mitch Albom teaches us how to talk to those who are slowly going downhill and shows us how to celebrate their lives in his book, *Tuesdays with Morrie* [20]. Susie, Charles, Mark, Jesse, and Morrie all died from their illnesses, but each did so with grace, while living well.

Through their remembrances and the patients I see daily, I continue to learn to live differently. I can better see the colors of my personal web of wellness. While I know that our webs will continually change and no two are the same, I would like to share with you some of the threads in my web and ask: What threads do you find woven into your web?

Threads of My Web

- Be grateful, especially for family; create ways to be together and express my love. Thanks, Holly.
- Laugh more, especially at myself. Thanks, Mark.
- Give my gifts, while pursuing my dreams. Thanks, Mavourneen.
- Ask more questions; every person is my teacher. Thanks, Paul.

- Honor those whose shoulders I stand on; create daily reminders and tell more stories. Thanks, Bruce.
- Pursue spiritual growth; build on my Quaker roots. Thanks, Dad.
- Cook more for others; then spend more time at the kitchen table. Thanks, Fish.
- Push the limits, just some of the time. Thanks, Hallie.
- Learn to dance. Thanks, Mom.
- Remember always, what is—IS! Thanks, Joy.

Do you find, as I do, that the lessons of life seem more insightful or meaningful, and carry more weight when they are written down and bound in a cover? If so, I suggest that you follow Joy's example, get your own bound notebook, and begin to compose your own Top Ten List in a way that would impress even David Letterman.

STEP OUT OF THE BOX OF YOUR ILLNESS

"Stepping Out of the Box" is Joy's metaphor for making sure she takes the opportunity to challenge herself and build her confidence by doing something meaningful and joyful, even if it seems beyond her capabilities. When Joy attended her high school reunion she learned that the rewards justified the risks, so she was willing to pay the price that followed this experience, even the deep, persistent pain and fatigue of chronic illness. In exchange, she benefited from her alertness of anticipation, her youthful play with old friends, and the temporary silencing of her pain. How do you step out of the box of being sick? Have you learned to find pleasure and playfulness in spite of your illness? Even for those who are not ill, so much time is spent pursuing professional, personal, and do-good goals that having fun may get lost in the shuffle.

When I find myself doing this, I try to remember a thought that is written in my mother's book of daily reminders, "People who think having fun is a waste of time don't realize that playing involves a genuine investment of the self." There is a guaranteed return on this investment—it is a gift to those around you, and you WILL have fun!

Stepping out of the box requires taking a first step, and usually, this is the hardest one. In my office, I have a quote that I sometimes pass out to those who are ready for this step. It is from a book written by William Hutchinson Murray in 1951, *The Scottish Himalayan Expedition*, where he references Goethe:

> *Until one is committed, there is hesitancy, the chance to draw back. Concerning all acts of initiative (and creation), there is one elementary truth, the ignorance of which kills countless ideas and splendid plans: that the moment one definitely commits oneself, then Providence moves too. All sorts of things occur to help one that would never otherwise have occurred. A whole stream of events issues from the decision, raising in one's favor all manner of unforeseen incidents and meetings and material assistance, which no man could have dreamed would have come his way. Whatever you can do, or dream you can do, begin it. Boldness has genius, power and magic in it. Begin it now. [21]*

Or as the current day Nike slogan more succinctly suggests, *Just Do It.*

LEARN FROM KITCHEN TABLE WISDOM

Sometime ago I stepped away from my busy practice to take a much-needed trip to my family roots in the Midwest. This trip home would prove to be more than a restful time for me. It would be a nurturing time where my old memories and new feelings could bubble and blend together. The grace Joy describes in her stories helped me see more keenly and listen more deeply to the everyday experiences of my home and family. My web of wellness was brightened and strengthened. It helped me see more clearly the many threads of different colors that hold the web together. Let me describe.

The visit began with a rare, unplanned day with my mother—no agenda, no list, no chores. First, we enjoyed a sunrise breakfast on her cozy deck, overlooking her small, beautiful backyard garden. A youthful bunny rabbit, his antenna ears alert, joined us. While he blissfully munched on ground cover, I crunched granola and we all shared the ambiance and early morning light. After breakfast Mom and I walked around the neighborhood and I listened to her running commentary on landscape design, the variety of climbing plants and flowers, her walking friend from grammar school, the neighborhood bridge group, and the community naysayer.

We arrived at the local coffee shop to meet the Monday Morning Ladies Who Drink (Coffee). Coffee table wisdom is much like kitchen table wisdom, except at the kitchen table mothers tell children what needs to be, while at the coffee table grandmothers tell friends how it really is. On this day, topics included the prognosis for future vacation care of grandchildren (Never again!), the humorous acknowledgment of each other's idiosyncrasies, and the discount airfares that invite the next opportunity for stepping out. I recognized that this kind of simple sharing is what nurtures the immune system, and fills the heart.

Later, at a neighborhood café, I met its owner, Scott, father of seven boys. When the old train track was converted into a bicycle trail and the train depot came up for sale, Scott moved to realize a dream. He gave up his law practice and bought the building, converting it into a family restaurant and coffee shop. Scott's dream of owning a restaurant fed into his dream of desiring more family time, so the restaurant included a room full of toys and gym equipment for kids when they stop by with their moms after a morning walk. Scott's own young boys are often found there and his older sons work with him. Regulars, my mom included, have become part of their extended family. The place overflowed with a sense of community and well-being.

The next day we drove to my wife's hometown, where Peg, my sister-in-law, gave me the book, *Kitchen Table Wisdom* [2]. The next morning I took it outside for some early morning reading and thinking, passing through the kitchen where my mother-in-law, Nana, sat at her old round oak table and dispensed her own kitchen table wisdom about the Greatest Generation, hers, of course. While she and my wife spoke of commitment, sacrifice and honor, I sat at my quiet garden table next to a bowl of red, sun-ripening tomatoes and watched the rising sun as it burned through the dust-filled air of the cornfields and turned the August sky a brilliant orange. Just as the morning cricket serenade began, I re-entered the kitchen to the familiar sound of Nana's roaring, infectious laugh, which meant she has just told her daughter a funny story on herself.

Nana seemed to sense that I had much on my mind and changed the subject, saying, "I think losing confidence is the biggest problem when people get old." She shared some of her own favorite confidence-building activities—driving fast, mowing her own lawn on a small tractor, and working long hours in her garden. Then she recalled a friend who had just recovered from a bout of shingles and shared another message that dovetailed with my own concerns. "It forced her to slow down and think. It is so easy to forget to be grateful." When Nana and my wife moved on to an analysis of our three sons, I took the opportunity to get up for another bowl of fresh peaches and blueberries, and returned to the deck thinking about Nana's insights about being sick and living well, maintaining confidence and being grateful.

DISCOVER AND GIVE YOUR GIFTS

Joy's Top Ten List includes the instruction "Find a way to share your gifts." I saw a beautiful example of this during a recent trip to Tennessee. I attended a dinner, hosted by the Arthritis Foundation and the local rheumatology group, at Nashville's famous Bluebird Café, the birthplace of many new Country-and-Western talents. In the center of the small diner, four musicians sat in the round, playing and singing. The energy flowing between the performers and the audience was palpable. One woman, who played the guitar and sang beautifully, shared with us that she pulled the group together as thanks for the treatment and care she had received from her local rheumatologist. The gifts she received from her doctor had encouraged her to invite these musicians to join her in offering their own gifts of music and fun.

I recently took dance lessons and learned another truth about giving gifts—it doesn't take more than showing up, smiling, and doing your best. As Pooh points out, one may be limited by thinking too hard about what you have to give or what talents you want to share. Unlike Joy, I do not feel at all natural while dancing. I was a tall gangly kid and hid out among the chairs or in the corners during school dances. When I was in junior high, my Mom sent me to a dance school, but it still felt awkward. As an adult, I again tried lessons a couple of times. I set my jaw, tried too hard, and never relaxed or had fun. My wife, Holly, therefore, didn't have fun either, since I was the one who was supposed to lead, while she tried to follow. It finally dawned on me that a gift I could give my wife was to take dance lessons on my own, so I could learn how to lead effectively. Then I would invite her to join me.

In the class, I found that laughing at my flubs was also a gift to other men who were just as uptight as I used to be. And for those designated to be the followers, usually the women in the class, I gave two gifts. I made them look good, and I was better than a broom. I am sure I also helped them to be more patient with their partners who were also still learning to lead. My gift to myself, to my wife, and to the class was just trying my best and having fun, no matter what.

REMEMBER THAT IT IS NEVER TOO LATE FOR HOPE AND CHANGE

I would like to conclude our journey together by sharing a poem written by my niece, Annie. It is an important reminder of the power in each of us to return at any time to the wisdom of our mother's kitchen table or to the threads of our own web of wellness.

My niece Annie lived on the family farm in Indiana, down the road from Nana. A few months after my trip back home, Annie was on her way to a gathering at her church. She pulled out onto a highway in the glare of the afternoon sun and was killed in a car accident. I had a chance to read a journal that Annie's third grade teacher had encouraged her to start, and that Annie continued for several years. I would like to close with Annie's simple wisdom, in her own words and spelling, from that journal.

Never Too Late
by Annie Horton
Age 8
Your shouldn't think its too late to ride on a hoarse,
Because its never too late.
Its not too late to be happy.
Its not too late to cry.
Its never too late to do inything.
It will never beto late to light a lantern.
It will never beto late to love someone.

Life itself is a daily gift that can be interrupted at any time. So, join me in enjoying a sunrise breakfast of peaches and berries while you take a moment to appreciate your past journey and all that is to come. I hope you have found your own wisdom and comfort through our stories. Good luck in weaving your web of wellness.

Chronic Illness Care: In the Eye of the Storm

We have asked Dr. Robert Crittenden to address some questions about the Affordable Care Act, an important concern to individuals with chronic illness. Dr. Crittenden, MD, MPH, is a primary care physician and health policy expert from the University of Washington and is the Executive Director of the Herndon Alliance, a coalition of over 200 organizations focused on ensuring all Americans have affordable high quality care.

Since the first edition of this book, a lot has transpired to potentially improve the care available for people with chronic illnesses. Buffeted by one of the most partisan battles in years, the Affordable Care Act passed the House and Senate and was signed into law in 2010. It is now being reviewed by the Supreme Court. While the Supreme Court may decide in a number of different ways, the underlying problems we face will continue, no matter what the decisions. A lot has been said about the act that is false and much that is hyperbole. The truth, as always, lies between. In Dr. Crittenden's opinion, there is more potential benefit for people with chronic illnesses in this law than in any change, public or private, in health care policy in the past 50 years. Up until now, the trends have all been going the wrong way.

We appreciate his willingness to help us become better informed, so that we all can become better advocates for those who live with chronic illness.

HOW AND WHY HAS OUR INSURANCE-BASED HEALTH CARE SYSTEM LIMITED COMPREHENSIVE, CHRONIC ILLNESS CARE?

We have a health care system that is rooted in history and is slow to come to terms with our lives and diseases. For over 500 years, physicians and health care workers have had license to treat the body, but only in the past 100 years have mind and spirit issues been part of the scope of health care—and then only with baggage, blame, and limits. The vestiges of that are found in the health coverage we have had up to the very recent past that always limited the care for mental and spiritual health while fully supporting physical health interventions. The recently passed laws that provide parity for mental health have helped, but there remain limits to integrating the full range of services that are needed if chronic conditions are to be treated well and people with chronic conditions are supported so they can live as well as possible. Chronic care requires integration of many different services that are well identified, but rarely functionally coordinated. The parity laws are a rare bright spot in the care for people with chronic conditions, but this improvement has been undercut by the rapid changes in the insurance industry.

Up until the 1970s, many nonprofit insurers "community rated," that is, they provided insurance for everyone for the same cost. They felt that it was their duty to offer the same rates to everyone who bought their insurance, so people who had illnesses paid the same as healthy people. During the 70s they succumbed to the competition from for-profit insurers. When for-profit insurers entered local markets, they aimed for the healthy populations and tried to avoid those with chronic conditions as they could charge the healthy people less, attract them away from community rated insurers and still make a handsome profit. This change in the market began a race to the bottom and the chronically ill were excluded whenever possible.

WHAT ARE SOME OTHER REASONS PATIENTS DON'T HAVE ACCESS TO INSURANCE COVERAGE?

Insurance companies have a responsibility to maximize profits for their shareholders. It is their fiduciary responsibility. A shameful period in our history began where we sliced and diced insurance coverage for employers, individuals, and families. The old and the sick were priced out of coverage unless they had a protector—an employer or the government making sure they had affordable coverage. Large employers had enough clout to negotiate the lowest prices with insurers and they included all of their employees and their dependents. The federal government provided Medicare for people over 65 and the chronically disabled. The federal and state governments teamed up to provide coverage through Medicaid for poor children, their mothers (not fathers or childless women), poor seniors, blind people, and the temporarily disabled. This latter program pays for the bulk of nursing home care for many of our elderly relatives. But, if you do not fit into any of those categories, and especially if you lose your job, you have little or no protection. The spike in bankruptcies due to health care costs is the tip of this iceberg.

WHAT ROLE HAVE INSURANCE COMPANIES PLAYED IN RISING HEALTH CARE COSTS?

Insurance companies have had few tools and little interest in constraining health care costs. In the early 1990s there was a lot of talk about insurance companies managing care and controlling costs. They entered into ill-fated efforts to control costs with no skills, expertise, or understanding of how to improve quality and reduce costs. The 1990s debacle of "managed care" came from those amateur efforts. Organizations that actually knew how to improve quality and decrease costs were tarred with the same brush. Organizations like the Mayo Clinic, Kaiser Health Plans, and Geisinger Clinic have excelled and have demonstrated ways to improve quality and control costs but most commercial insurers failed.

After the flirtation with managed care, insurance companies returned to the methods they knew well. They worked to improve their profitability by excluding individuals and companies that had high risks. Theoretically, insurance companies should be in a position to integrate, coordinate, and use financial and other levers to improve the care for people with chronic conditions. They made failed efforts to accomplish these tasks and reverted back to managing risks (avoiding sick people) rather than improving care. Costs have increased and chronic care has suffered.

WHY IS CHRONIC ILLNESS CARE SO IMPORTANT AND SUCH A CHALLENGE TO OUR CURRENT SYSTEM?

Chronic conditions are the biggest challenge to our current health care, and particularly in the future, as many more people age. People with chronic diseases and conditions consume 70% of our health costs. Our poor health rating internationally has a number of causes, but the biggest is our failure to prevent, treat, and rehabilitate people with chronic conditions. We have successful models of intense, integrated, team approaches for the frail elderly. We have examples of intensive outpatient care—again in teams—for high-risk children and adults. We have examples of team approaches to primary care populations that have demonstrated improved quality and decreased costs. These all are win–win opportunities for the chronically ill, but, these are exceptions and not the rule.

Some employers, insurance companies, hospitals and physicians see improved care as their responsibility, but most feel they cannot move ahead with the needed improvements. They say, "If the insurance company would pay for the costs of the changes," "if the physicians would all join into large groups," or "if doctors worked for hospitals" there could be change. There is hesitancy to take the first step—no one wants to be first and an outlier. Inaction is safer for many institutions and providers. To get a broad movement toward improved care, we all need a commitment to take the first step.

WHAT IS THE BACKGROUND TO THE AFFORDABLE CARE ACT STRATEGY?

During the past ten years, there has been interest by employers, providers and government policy makers in improving the quality and outcomes of the health system. There are bright spots around the country where private, public and joint public–private efforts have been undertaken to improve quality, integrate and coordinate care, and improve outcomes. These efforts have focused on a number of approaches:

1. Some have been focused on information technology as a backbone to best practices, integration, and quality improvement.
2. Some have involved data collection to provide feedback and enable incentives to be developed.
3. Some have used active participation in purchasing in a geographical area to bring consistent incentives into play, encouraging physicians, hospitals, and other providers to improve their systems and care.
4. And, some have developed teams of providers working together with the dual goal of improving care and decreasing costs.

There are successes in all of these areas and the most successful have used combinations of the above. The work done to improve concepts of primary care, develop intensive treatment systems for sick and expensive populations, improve care provided in hospitals, and integrate prevention, primary care, and hospital care have been instructive. We now have guidelines about how we can improve care and methods of system improvement that can be applied as we move forward. The work of the Institute for Healthcare Improvement, programs for the frail elderly, the efforts to refine, improve, and implement the Primary Care Medical Home are concrete examples of these important efforts.

We need to make these improvements available to all people with chronic conditions. The recent experiments are not enough, outcomes have not improved overall, costs have continued to spiral up, more people are falling through the cracks, and many are not getting the care they need.

When talking to everyday Americans, the vast majority report bad experiences with the health systems and cite similar problems like:

- Repetitively filling out forms asking for the same information at every facility they visit.
- Consulting doctors who are missing some of the records they need.
- Repetition of recent tests.
- Personal physicians who have not been informed of follow-up plans after hospital stays.
- Patient preference documents (like a living will) cannot be found, or if found, are not believed.

Then, there are those rare moments when someone recounts being in a health care system or community that is focused on the patient, communicates internally, provides real information, encourages patient participation in decisions about their care, and succeeds in serving the needs of the patient, family, and, sometimes, the whole community.

The challenge we have is to make this high quality and affordable care available to everyone in the country. We need to align our goals, incentives, systems, and providers so we are all focused on making the patient experience and quality care our prime focus. We all need to have the same goal. We need to take the best practices, encourage their continual improvement, and do all we can to move those best practices into use by many different providers and groups. No one size fits all, but we need to identify the best care for the people in a system or community. We need to develop a system that can make appropriate changes quickly, test those changes and refine them, and continually improve.

HOW IS THE AFFORDABLE CARE ACT AN IMPORTANT FIRST STEP?

The Affordable Care Act, the health reform law passed in 2010, is our national commitment to beginning this journey. The elements of that law are both sweeping and insufficient. We now have a commitment to ramp up prevention, integrate care, improve our services, measure our success, and begin the long road toward a more functional and successful health care system for all people in our country.

At the same time, much of the law is an outline, with questions that need answers. Those answers are simply not known now, but we can address many of our shortcomings and we can be successful if we use this law as a constructive first step. This law is an outline for change and many of the details will need to be filled in at the state and national levels over the next few years. States will need to pass laws, implement oversight activities, and address the needs of all of their residents to ensure the new law works for them. National leaders will need to listen to their constituents, and make incremental improvements for many years to come. And, most important, doctors, hospitals, health insurers, and other providers need to commit to broad and effective changes that include all people in our communities.

There has been a lot of partisanship in the development of this law, but we need to get beyond the political posturing and address real issues that people have. Contrary to the public discussion, much of the law is a melding of ideas from both parties. Given the great need people with chronic conditions have, it is time to roll our up our sleeves and make this law work. It needs improvements and those should be discussed with the goal of making our health care system work, not to serve partisan rhetoric about socialism or capitalism.

WHAT DOES THE AFFORDABLE CARE ACT DO TO MOVE US TOWARD A BETTER HEALTH SYSTEM FOR PEOPLE WITH CHRONIC ILLNESSES?

1. Emphasizes Prevention

The first change is a significant emphasis on prevention. Prevention is the rock on which we build the health of our families and future generations. Encouraging healthy behaviors and catching cancer at an early stage are effective ways to improve our health. Personal prevention is now included as a covered service in Medicare and will be in most health plans. This type of prevention is a personal service you get at a doctor's office and includes screening for cancer, cholesterol, and high blood pressure. These improve our health and well-being. Diseases are detected earlier at more easily treated stages. There is little evidence that these practices save money in the long run, but they definitely improve our health and happiness and enable us to live better longer.

The new health law also makes the largest investment in our lifetimes in an area called community prevention. This is the least sexy thing in health care, but has the greatest possibility of improving the health of our children, helping people function well during their lives, and enabling older people to function well as they age. This type of prevention removes barriers so people can choose the healthy behaviors we know work, such as being active, eating well, having safe water, avoiding injuries, and decreasing the stress of poverty, crime, and social dysfunction. This type of prevention is also the most difficult to support because it is seen as a personal responsibility, but it truly needs community action to succeed. It is in the interest of our children that we do succeed with this prevention.

At present, insurance companies have little incentive to invest now to prevent a disease that will save money in ten years. Community prevention requires local resources and local leadership to change the structures and environment we live in. Many communities lack the money to make the changes needed to enable people to walk more and eat better food. Providing funding for communities to voluntarily make investments in reducing the barriers to activity and good food is a wise investment. Costs are avoided, kids grow and learn better, families have more years to spend together and working people remain productive longer.

2. Makes Care More Affordable

The greatest concern for many people with chronic conditions is accessing affordable insurance. Often people get ill or are unable to function at work, lose their jobs, and, therefore, their employer-sponsored care. Or, a person may be able to work, but is fearful of starting his or her own business because of a pre-existing condition. Without the protection of a large employer plan, a chronically ill individual or small business owner will often find he or she cannot buy affordable insurance. Insurance companies often price chronically ill people out of the market. There are some government options, but they are limited and available now only for people in some narrow categories. You need to be totally disabled, aged, blind, a pregnant woman, or a child to get government support. Some programs like Medicare are open for everyone who is over 65 years of age or who are certified as disabled. People with Medicare are included in a large pool financed by payroll and general taxes and individual contributions. But not all people have access to this social insurance.

Some people in the private market with chronic conditions have to go to high-risk pools—small programs in states that provide insurance for people otherwise excluded from insurance because they have pre-existing medical conditions. These small plans are expensive. For over a third of applicants, the plans are unaffordable and so they go without coverage. Insurance companies do many things that are legal in order to avoid insuring sick people.

The new Affordable Care Act changes this. It ensures that children and adults with medical conditions cannot be excluded from private insurance. It provides a process where states can establish standards for benefits so appropriate services are available to all patients including physical, mental health, and preventive services. It also establishes local marketplaces, called exchanges, that will enable people without coverage or those changing coverage to voluntarily shop, compare, and buy health insurance. And, most importantly, there will be health insurance available to all people in the state at an affordable price through that marketplace. All people will have to pay what they can, but there will be support for lower income people so they can buy an affordable insurance product.

3. Improves Coordination of Care

The new health law provides support for local physicians and other providers to work together in teams and improve the health of their patients. There is ample evidence that health providers can improve the quality of care, improve patient satisfaction, record measurable improvements in health outcomes, and decrease the cost of care, but few doctors and their support teams are working at this high level of functioning now. Personally they are functioning well, but as a system they are functioning poorly. The new health law supports and accelerates changes that many doctors, nurses, hospitals, and insurers are making to improve the care they provide so it is more coordinated and effective.

4. Improves Care for Frail Patients

The small group of patients with many chronic problems who, without support, would be institutionalized is the most expensive group to care for. These patients desperately want to remain at home. There are a number of programs around the country that mobilize a wide variety of resources to support independent living for these people. These programs are able to keep people at home, out of hospitals, and more able to live and enjoy life. They also have been shown to save overall costs. For years there has been resistance to undertaking these efforts, partially from the risk of undertaking the responsibility for this population and partially from the crazy patchwork of funding that goes toward support for these patients. Medical care, home care, pharmaceuticals, housing, transportation, and other support services are usually funded separately and from different insurers and agencies. Bringing all of this funding into one pool so that the services can be coordinated and appropriate for that patient is a trick that most institutions cannot accomplish.

The new law has focused on these patients and is developing best practices, enabling federal and state funds from multiple sources to be pooled and is changing the rules that now block successful intensive use of services that these people need. All patients want to remain at home when the alternative is an institution. This concept is truly a win–win.

WHAT NEEDS TO BE DONE IN OUR COMMUNITIES TO MAKE OUR HEALTH SYSTEMS RESPONSIVE TO PATIENT NEEDS?

This law is a work in progress. It builds on the hard work that has been done for years by many people trying to make our health system better. Little in this law is new; rather, this is the largest and most coordinated effort to implement proven improvements in our health system. But, without your participation, we will not have the results we deserve and need. The gains that people with chronic diseases will accrue from this law depend on continual improvements at the federal level and implementation at the state level. Federal policymakers—your representatives—need to understand that they must continually work with you, listen to you, and respond with appropriate policies that work for people with chronic conditions. As with any new policy, and particularly one that interfaces with such a complicated health system, there will be missteps and complications. These are expected. You are at the front line and you need to identify problems and potential improvements as the law is implemented.

One example is the insurance exchange, a voluntary marketplace where patients can get affordable insurance when they change employment or enter the insurance market. People will be able to make apples-to-apples comparisons and shop for the insurance that is right for them. The details—who runs it, what benefits are covered, and how you can access this insurance—are dependent on state policy makers. Your experience is what the policy makers want and need to know. Without your input, insurance companies will have a lot to say, and that may or may not be in your best interests as a patient. You need to be working with your associations and representatives making sure these structures live up to their potential. But changes in policy are only a small part of the needed change.

WHAT ADVOCACY DO OUR READERS NEED TO UNDERTAKE TO MAKE SURE THE HEALTH SYSTEM MAKES POSITIVE CHANGES THAT ARE GOOD FOR THEM, THEIR FAMILIES, AND THEIR FRIENDS WITH CHRONIC ILLNESS?

The most fundamental and important changes for people with chronic illnesses will happen at doctors' offices, hospitals, and other local care sites. To effectively construct functional and coordinated teams where your physicians and other providers can work, provide you with the highest quality care, and ensure your health is as good as possible, many providers will need to change the way they organize and provide care. This continuation of changes is underway in many sites and spreading into the broader system. There have already been remarkable improvements in patient satisfaction, improvements in quality of care and decreases in cost, but if these changes are to be done appropriately, there needs to be patient input into the improvements and feedback about changes as they are made. Changes in systems need to be focused on the people with chronic illnesses and your participation and input will be needed.

SUMMARY

The largest change in health policy for the past 50 years—the Affordable Care Act—is an opportunity, but any large change of this type cannot be successful if left only to policy makers, health insurers, and health care professionals. The people who have the biggest stake in the potential changes are those with chronic diseases. We know these changes can work, but only if patients get a place at the table and ensure that the changes work for all of us.

Reflection

As Dr. Overman and I were completing the first edition of *You Don't LOOK Sick!*, my husband and I moved from our rural, island home in Washington State to Austin, Texas, the state where I was born and spent my childhood. We thought the warm, dry climate would be better for me, and it has proven to be. It also seems that my immune system reacts less to this environment, the one that I grew up in. We thought I would have easier access to medical care here, and I do, but I had to find all new doctors, and I don't have Dr. Overman to treat me anymore. When we renewed our writing partnership for the second edition, I renewed my appreciation for Dr. Overman's sympathetic and caring approach. He has lived our principles in his practice for years now. He has greater confidence in the opportunities presented by utilizing a phase model to treat chronic illness. His anecdotes, stories, and lessons all come from a deep well of personal experience. This wisdom is his gift, not only to our readers who are coping with illness, but also to the health care professionals who are treating them.

When we first moved to Texas, I felt so much better I thought perhaps my health was returning, but soon I began to have a new symptom, pain on the right side of my face, along my upper jaw. It seemed like it must be a dental issue and I spent three years enduring root canals, replacement fillings, even sinus surgery before my internist identified the problem by a process of elimination. The diagnosis was trigeminal neuralgia, a chronic inflammation of the huge, tree like nerve that runs along the side of the face and jaw. It is called the "worst pain known to science" and the "suicide disease." This paralyzing pain, untreated for years, truly took me to my knees. Once I finally found my neurologist and treatment began, I had to go back to the beginning—to the rage, the grief, the stingy acceptance, the submission, the making of peace.

But there was a silver lining. When my neurologist started me on an anti-seizure drug for the nerve pain, all my other symptoms improved and I was able to reduce medications overall.

After a few years, the medication was no longer effectively controlling my facial pain. We tried more medicine, and other combinations, but nothing worked. This condition, like other chronic conditions, also had many triggers—cold, heat, wind, vibration, barometric pressure changes, talking, singing, stress. In time, any increase in my heart rate exacerbated the pain. My world began to get very, very small. We had to look for other answers.

In November, 2010, I had brain surgery. It turned out, as my surgeon had believed, there were veins pressing on this trigeminal nerve, causing constant irritation and inflammation. The surgeon moved these veins aside and placed a tiny Teflon sponge over the nerve to act as a barrier. A year later, I was able to go off medication for this condition completely. My other diagnoses, interstitial cystitis, fibromyalgia, and mixed connective tissue disease remain well controlled.

Over the quarter century that I've lived with illness I have experienced many advances in treatment, from both the Western scientific community and from alternative therapies. Many have been effective for me. The result is that I am much improved. I have less pain, less fatigue, less brain fog, and take less medication. I laughingly tell my friends that I got old in my thirties. Now, in my sixties, I am getting younger all the time.

I share this story to give you hope. Dr. Overman and I wrote this book for patients enduring illnesses that cannot be cured, cannot even be seen. As one of those patients, I want to share my experience that, over time, a chronic condition can get much, much better and cures, like my successful brain surgery, may be possible. So my final word is, make peace, but don't give up hope. There is always hope.

DR. OVERMAN

My recurrent atrial fibrillation has been challenging, but I have stayed active and my rheumatology practice is better than ever. After leaving a large group practice, I started a solo practice and then helped found The Seattle Arthritis Clinic, where we now have seven rheumatologists, two counselors, a registered dietician, a nurse practitioner, and full ancillary services and a research program. This integrated practice has been tremendously rewarding to me personally and professionally, and I believe with this model we can better treat the many patients I see in all the different phases of their journeys.

Joy's ups and downs and my work with the counselors in the office remind me over and over again of a very important fact—the journey to *Living Well* is not a straight path, nor is it ever a final destination. The ups and downs of chronic illness are accompanied by re-cycling through the phases of coping over and over again: the crisis of new or aggravated problems; relearning how to manage symptoms; grief over past, current, or feared loss; and the feeling of wellness that returns like light at morning. These cycles are likely to recur not only with illness, but during other life crises as well. Days pass into seasons, and darkness and cold lead to the warmth of spring. Having shared our journey, we hope that now you can apply the lessons of the phases of illness and better weather all of life's challenges, including illness.

I would like to leave you with a morning prayer I found and memorized during one of the dark times of my brother's illness. I keep it next to the phone in my office, and still try to say it daily. It is found in the front of John O'Donohue's book, *Eternal Echoes: Exploring Our Yearning to Belong* [22]. May it remind you of the light that follows the dark, the quiet that nurtures you, the miracles of your body, and the grace-filled way to approach each day.

Matins

I.

Somewhere, out at the edges, the night
Is turning and the waves of darkness
Begin to brighten the shore of dawn.

The heavy dark falls back to earth
And the freed air goes wild with light,

The heart fills with fresh, bright breath
And thoughts stir to give birth to colour.

II.
I arise today

In the name of Silence
Womb of the Word,
In the name of Stillness
Home of Belonging,
In the name of the Solitude
Of the Soul and the Earth

I arise today

Blessed by all things,
Wings of breath,
Delight of eyes,
Wonder of whisper,
Intimacy of touch,
Eternity of soul,
Urgency of thought,
Miracle of health,
Embrace of God.

May I live this day

Compassionate of heart,
Gentle in word,
Gracious in awareness,
Courageous in thought,
Generous in love.

Bibliography

1. Fennell, Patricia A. 2003. *Managing Chronic Illness Using The Four-Phase Treatment Approach*. Hoboken, NJ: John Wiley and Sons Inc.

   Fennell, Patricia A. 2012. Revised Edition. *The Chronic Illness Workbook: Strategies and Solutions for Taking Back Your Life*. Albany, NY: Albany Health Publishing. (Previous edition: 2001. Oakland, CA: New Harbinger Publications, Inc.)

   Jason, Leonard A.; Fennell, Patricia A.; Taylor, Renee. 2003. *Handbook of Chronic Fatigue Syndrome and Fatiguing Illnesses*. Hoboken, NJ: John Wiley and Sons Inc.
2. Remen, Rachel. 1996. *Kitchen Table Wisdom: Stories That Heal*. New York: Riverhead Books.
3. Becker, Ernest. 1973. *The Denial of Death*. New York: The Free Press; London: Collier Macmillan.
4. Foster, Richard J. 1998. *Celebration of Discipline: The Path to Spiritual Growth*, 20th anniversary edition. New York, NY Harper.
5. Reid, T. R. 2009. *The Healing of America: A Global Quest for Better, Cheaper, and Fairer Health Care*. New York: The Penguin Press.
6. *King James Bible*, The Old Testament, Psalms 118:24.
7. *King James Bible*, The New Testament, Romans 8:28.
8. *The New International Bible Dictionary*. 1987. J. D. Douglas, Revising editor, Merrill C. Tenney, General Editor, Zondervan.

9. *Bartlett's Familiar Quotations*. 2002. 17th edition. Boston, MA: Little, Brown and Company.

10. L'Engle, Madeline. 2001. *Walking on Water: Reflections on Faith and Art*, Wheaton Literary Series, 5th edition. Colorado Springs, CO: WaterBrook Press, p. 27.

11. Turner, Dale. 1998. *Different Seasons: Twelve Months of Wisdom and Inspiration*, 1st edition. New Lenox, IL: High Tide Press.

12. Gruber, William. 2003. *Letting Go: A Memoir*. Bloomington, IN: iUniverse, Inc.

13. McElroy, Molly, 2011. "Less depression for working moms who expect that they 'can't do it all.'" *UW Today, News and Information*, August 22.

14. Easwaran, Eknath. The Blue Mountain Center for Meditation. http://www.easwaran.org/about-eknath-easwaran.html.

15. Lorig, Kate. 2000. *Living a Healthy Life with Chronic Conditions: Self-Management of Heart Disease, Arthritis, Diabetes, Asthma, Bronchitis, Emphysema & Others*. Berkeley, CA: Publishers Group West.

16. Bernhard, Toni. 2010. *How to Be Sick: A Buddhist-Inspired Guide for the Chronically Ill and Their Caregivers*. Somerville, MA: Wisdom Publications.

17. Edwards, Laurie. 2008. *Life Disrupted: Getting Real About Chronic Illness in Your Twenties and Thirties*. New York, NY: Walker & Company.

18. Hoff, Benjamin. 1983. *Tao of Pooh*. New York, NY: Penguin Books (Non-Classics).

19. Albom, Mitch. 1997. *Tuesdays with Morrie: An Old Man, a Young Man, and Life's Greatest Lesson*. New York, NY: Doubleday.

20. Murray, William Hutchinson. 1951. The Scottish Himalayan Expedition. http://german.about.com/library/blgermyth12.htm.

21. O'Donohue's, John. 1999. *Eternal Echoes: Exploring Our Yearning to Belong*. New York, NY: Cliff Street Books Harper Collins.

Resources

Most medical conditions have an associated organization or informational arm. Abundant helpful resources for patients are available through web searches using key words of illnesses or symptoms. For those who do not yet have a clear diagnosis, there are general medical sites with search engines that will match symptoms to medical conditions. Also, there are sites to help patients cope with particular symptoms, such as chronic pain. Once diagnosed, patients can find help and support in managing illness and accessing care through illness support and research organizations. Almost every site provides additional resources through recommendations or an online store. We list below sites that we have found helpful.

GENERAL MEDICAL WEBSITES

The web has become the world's largest source for medical information. Reputable sites can be excellent starting points for someone with a diagnosis and many questions. By searching each site, you can find summary information about your issues. Use caution, though, especially in chat rooms and other unmonitored forums. Information in these forums are anecdotal and may be misleading or totally wrong. Here are some recommended sites:

CDC.gov: The Centers for Disease Control and Prevention's site, with searchable information and statistics on many health topics, including arthritis.

Health.nih.gov: From the National Institutes of Health (NIH), a very comprehensive site with information about clinical trials, drug evaluations, and disease-specific therapies, in addition to general topics.

ImprovingChronicCare.org: Site sponsored by Edward Wagner and the Robert Wood Johnson Foundation to help organizations interested in improving chronic care management.

ASKJAN.org: The Job Accommodation Network provides help with questions about workplace accommodations and the Americans with Disabilities Act (ADA) or related legislation.

MayoClinic.com: Mayo Clinic's consumer site, offering health and medical information, self-improvement strategies, and disease management tools.

Medlineplus.gov: Another comprehensive site from the NIH with a medical encyclopedia, medical dictionary, recent medical news, and drug and health information.

NCCAM.nih.gov: This site, from the National Center for Complementary and Alternative Medicine, lists alerts and advisories about treatments and medications. It also offers information about alternative medicine and links to conventional medical topics and information.

Psychiatry.org: The American Psychiatric Association is the world's largest psychiatric organization representing more than 36,000 psychiatric physicians from the United States and around the world.

APA.org: The American Psychological Association is the U.S. scientific and professional organization representing psychology.

Quackwatch.com: As the name implies, this site offers information about health fraud and current concerns about medications and treatments. It lists consumer protection agencies and services and includes comments about questionable services, websites, advertisements, and products, as well as non-recommended sources of health advice.

WebMD.com: A comprehensive, searchable site that offers information for the newly diagnosed, expert advice, and extensive general health resources.

DISEASE-SPECIFIC ASSOCIATIONS AND WEBSITES

This list only begins to scratch the surface of the web-based help available for patients with specific invisible chronic illnesses. Many of our readers first found *You Don't LOOK Sick* through a review or recommendation on a disease specific website. Those marked with an asterisk (*) represent organizations that, at a national or regional level, have invited the authors to speak or conduct a workshop. Many also reviewed or recommended our book. We have arranged them alphabetically by disease or symptom.

*APS Foundation of America (Antiphospholipid Antibody Syndrome)
PO Box 801
LaCrosse, WI 54602-0801
www.apsfa.org

American Cancer Society
National Home Office
250 Williams Street NE
Atlanta, GA 30303
(800) 227-2345
www.cancer.org

*American Chronic Pain Association
PO Box 850
Rocklin, CA 95677
(919) 632-3208
(800) 533-3231
www.theacpa.org

*Arthritis Foundation
PO Box 7669
Atlanta, GA 30357-0669
(800) 283-7800
www.arthritis.org

*CFIDS Association (Chronic Fatigue Syndrome)
PO Box 220398
Charlotte, NC 28222
(704) 365-2343
www.cfids.org

Bent but Not Broken: Providing Emotional, Educational & Financial Resources to Patients & Their Caretakers Living With CFIDS/CFS
www.bentbutnotbroken.org

Co Cure ME/CFS and Fibromyalgia Information Exchange
Cooperate and Communicate for a Cure
www.co-cure.org

Crohn's and Colitis Foundation
386 Park Avenue South, 17th Floor
New York, NY 10016
(800) 932-2423
www.ccfa.org

*The National Fibromyalgia Association
2121 S. Towne Centre Place, Suite 300
Anaheim, CA 92806
(714) 921-0150
www.fmaware.org

*Fibromyalgia Network
PO Box 31750
Tucson, AZ 85751
(800) 853-2929
www.fmnetnews.com

*Gastroparesis Patient Association for Cures and Treatments
702 Winebary Circle
Lewisberry, PA 17339
1-888-URG-PACT
www.g-pact.org

National Headache Foundation
820 N. Orleans, Suite 411
Chicago, IL 60610
(888) 643-5552
www.headaches.org

*Interstitial Cystitis Association
1760 Old Meadow Road, Suite 500
Maclean, VA 22102
(703) 442-2070
www.ichelp.org

Lupus Foundation of America
2000 L Street N.W. Suite 410
Washington, DC 20036
(800) 558-0121 (information request line)
(202) 349-1155 (main office)
www.lupus.org

*Lyme Disease Association
PO Box 1438
Jackson, NJ 08527
(888) 366-6611
www.lymediseaseassocation.org

*The Mastocytosis Society
PO Box 129
Hastings, NE 68902-0129
www.tmsforacure.org

*MPN Education Foundation (myeloproliferative neoplasms)
PO Box 4758
Scottsdale, AZ 85261
www.mpninfo.org

*Myasthenia Gravis Foundation of America
355 Lexington Avenue, 15th Floor
New York, NY 10017
(800) 541-5454
www.myasthenia.org

The Myositis Association (TMA)
1737 King Street, Suite 600
Alexandria, VA 22314
(800) 821-7356
www.myositis.org

National Multiple Sclerosis Society
733 Third Avenue
New York, NY 10017
(800) 344-4867
www.nmss.org

*National Neutropenia Network
PO Box 1693
Brighton, Michigan 48116-5493
www.neutropenianet.org

*The Neuropathy Association, Inc.
60 East 42nd Street, Suite 942
New York, NY 10165
Tel: 212-692-0662
www.neuropathy.org

National Osteoporosis Foundation
1150 17th Street NW, Suite 850
Washington, DC 20036
(800) 231-4222
www.nof.org

Chronic Pain Anonymous
P.O. Box 107
Lutherville, MD 21094
www.chronicpainanonymous.org

*Parkinson's Disease Foundation
1359 Broadway, Suite 1509
New York, NY 10018
(212) 923-4700
www.pdf.org

*Scleroderma Foundation
300 Rosewood Drive, Suite 105
Danvers, MA 01923
(800) 722-HOPE (4673)
www.scleroderma.org

American Sickle Cell Anemia Association
DD Building at the Cleveland Clinic
10900 Carnegie Avenue
Cleveland, OH 44106
(216) 229-8600
www.ascaa.org

*Sjögren's Syndrome Foundation
6707 Democracy Blvd, Suite 325
Bethesda, MD 20817
(800) 475-6473
www.sjogrens.com

Spondylitis Association of America
16360 Roscoe Blvd, Suite 100
Van Nuys, CA 91406
(800) 777-8189
www.spondylitis.org

American Thyroid Association
6066 Leesburg Pike, Suite 550
Falls Church, VA 22041
(800) THYROID
www.thyroid.org

The Vasculitis Foundation
PO Box 28660
Kansas City, MO 64188-8660
(800) 277-9474
www.vasculitisfoundation.org

ONLINE NEWSLETTERS

Another source of information for patients is online newsletters. These may address a specific symptom or illness. They may also have a retail function and/or membership requirements. However, the summary of news and research that they offer can be helpful to patients trying to keep abreast of progress in medical research on the causes of illness, diagnostic tests, and the latest treatment options.

ProHealth: www.prohealth.com
This newsletter is subtitled "commerce with compassion" and publishes recent research on fibromyalgia and chronic fatigue and also markets vitamins and supplements.

Fibromyalgia Network: www.fmnetnews.com
This newsletter is dedicated to fibromyalgia treatment and research news. They do not accept advertisements, endorsements or pharmaceutical company grants.

ICA Update—ICAeNews: www.ichelp.org
The *ICA Update* is an award-winning quarterly magazine from the Interstitial Cystitis Association with in-depth stories about interstitial cystitis (IC) research, treatment, and lifestyle issues. The *ICA Update* is a benefit of membership in the Interstitial Cystitis Association (ICA). Donors who make an annual gift of $45 or more to the ICA also receive this unique magazine.

Discussion Questions for Patient Support Groups

We offer the following questions to help stimulate more a personal discussion about the topics raised in our book.

INTRODUCTION

- What stage are you experiencing in your illness journey: Getting Sick, Being Sick, Grief and Acceptance, or Living Well?
- How do you know?

GETTING SICK

Snake in the Mist

- Do you have a feeling that there is a snake in the mist?
- What is frightening to you about your illness?
- Which is most frightening, your present challenges or the unknown?

Three Strikes

- What would, or has, caused you to call a strike on a doctor?
- What are the qualities essential to you in your health care partner?

Pills, Procedures, and Paperwork

- Do you have a story from your own experience with insurers?
- What did you learned from the experience?
- What are the secrets to winning a claim?
- Have you had any embarrassing moments with illness that make you laugh now?

The Stuck Car

- Are you stuck in the ditch?
- How do you need to drive differently?
- In what ways have you realized your mind and body are connected?
- Do you have a team to help teach you and support your efforts?

BEING SICK

Pain

- What does your pain prevent you from doing?
- How do you effectively manage your pain?
- How does your pain affect others around you?

Disabled, But Not Invalid

- Have you ever been treated as if you were a fraud because you are ill?
- How did you handle it then?
- How might you handle it differently today?

The Ladies Who Lunch

- What are the five most thoughtless remarks people have made to you about being sick?
- How did you handle them?
- How did you feel afterward?
- How might you handle it differently now, so you maintain your peace of mind?

The Athlete and the Coach

- Is your primary doctor an effective coach?
- Are you the best athlete you can be?
- Are there elements of your physical, emotional, or spiritual training that need to be addressed for you to reach peak performance?
- How are you learning to make peace without giving up?

GRIEF AND ACCEPTANCE

I Cry

- What losses do you grieve from your life before illness?
- What makes you cry, or why don't you cry?

Still Time

- Has your illness allowed you to discover still time?
- Describe your place of peace.
- What interrupts your ability to achieve stillness or peacefulness?

A Gift of Grace

- How would you define grace?
- What examples can you share of the grace that has come to you through illness?
- What is the meaning of your illness for you, and how has it changed over time?

The Waves of Loss

- Can you recall a time when the rogue wave knocked you down?
- How did you get back up again?
- What has helped you find acceptance of your illness?
- Have you begun to build a new life with illness?

LIVING WELL

Joy's Top Ten List for Living Well, Even While Sick

- What is #1 on your top ten ways to live well even while sick?
- Has your #1 changed over time?
- What else on your list has helped you to live well?

Stepping Out of the Box

- Have you stepped out of the box lately?
- What did (would you like) to do?
- Was it (would it be) worth the price?

Natural High

- If you were to share one valuable lesson learned from illness, what would it be?

Weaving the Web of Wellness

- Who are the people who help you weave a web of wellness in your life?
- Can you name a few of the threads of your web?
- Do you have kitchen table wisdom to share?
- Have you found gifts you can give now?
- How has this helped you to feel better?

REFLECTIONS

- What kind of changes have you made in your lifestyle or treatment that makes you hopeful that the future can be better for you?

Index